beauty
pearls
for
chemo
girls

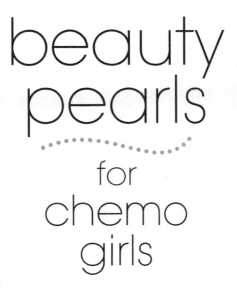

beauty pearls
for chemo girls

Marybeth Maida and Debbie Kiederer

Foreword by Betsey Johnson

CITADEL PRESS
Kensington Publishing Corp
www.kensingtonbooks.com

CITADEL PRESS BOOKS are published by

Kensington Publishing Corp.
119 West 40th Street
New York, NY 10018

All Kensington titles, imprints, and distributed lines are available at special quantity discounts for bulk purchases for sales promotions, premiums, fund-raising, educational, or institutional use. Special book excerpts or customized printings can also be created to fit specific needs. For details, write or phone the office of the Kensington special sales manager: Kensington Publishing Corp., 119 West 40th Street, New York, NY 10018, attn: Special Sales Department: phone 1-800-221-2647.

First printing: September 2009

10   9   8   7   6   5   4   3   2   1

Printed in the United States of America

Library of Congress Control Number: 2009923870

ISBN-13: 978-0-8065-3118-2
ISBN-10: 0-8065-3118-5

For Bruce, my husband, my love, my dearest friend:
When I was anything but beautiful, you never made me feel
anything but beautiful.

Your girl always,
Marybeth

For my cousin Karen Longo Leschke and my college roommate,
Susan Hauser Alexander, whom I will admire always for their
courage and perseverance as they battled their cancers—
may this book hold your memory forever.

And for my husband, Bobby Cucullo, who continues to be
my inspiration and the wind beneath my wings . . .

With great love,
Debbie

CONTENTS

Foreword *by Betsey Johnson*   **xiii**

Prologue   **1**

Our Panel of Experts   *1*
Survivors' Stories   *11*

Chapter 1. The Power of Makeup   **27**

Looking Good/Feeling Better   *28*
Why It Still Matters   *31*

Chapter 2. The Mane Event   **33**

First Things First—Buy a Wig   *36*
Choosing a Wig?   *38*
Synthetic or Human—Let's See What's Best   *39*
Insurance   *40*
Comfort + Style = Your Best Choice in Caps,
    Color, and Cut   *41*
Measuring for a Custom Wig   *45*
When the Wig Won't Work   *47*
Scarf-Tying Options   *48*

When the Shedding Starts   *54*
Caring for Your Scalp   *54*
Chemo Curls and Transitioning Back from
   Baldness   *55*
Finding Your Hair Helper   *57*

Chapter 3. Skin Deep   **61**

The Basics—Cleansing, Moisturizing,
   Protecting   *65*
Cleansing Your Face   *66*
. . . and Your Body   *67*
Moisturizing Your Face   *68*
. . . and Your Body   *69*
To Peel or Not to Peel—Exfoliation, Toners, and
   Astringents   *70*
Protecting Your Skin from the Sun   *72*
Hello, Face!   *73*
   Step 1: Look in the Mirror   *74*
      Foundation   *75*
      Concealer   *78*
      Blush   *79*
      Lips   *80*
   Step 2: All About Eyes   *81*
      Lashes   *81*
      Going False   *82*
      Brows   *84*
      Drawing on Brows   *85*
      Applying a Stencil   *86*
      Tints   *86*
      Sunken Eyes   *87*
      Dark Circles   *87*
   Step 3: Dealing with Skin-Related Side Effects   *88*
      Sallowness   *88*
      Ashiness   *89*

Redness/Flushing   *90*
Acne   *91*
Uneven Pigmentation   *92*
Rashes   *93*
Sunburn-like Pain   *94*
Neuropathy   *95*
Excessive Melanin   *95*
Keeping Your Sunny Side Up   *96*

Chapter 4. Chemo Style   **99**

What to Do   *102*
Laying the Foundation   *104*
Chemo Style—It's in the Eyes   *105*
. . . and the Size   *106*
All About Proportions   *108*
In the Eye of the Beholder   *109*
All About Accessories   *111*
Cottoning to Your Clothes   *115*
Hide and No One Will Seek   *116*
Excessive Thinness   *117*
Altered Skin Tone   *119*
The Finishing Touches—Hats and Scarves   *120*
Marilyn Monroe in the Park   *122*

Chapter 5. The Business of You   **125**

Selecting Your Medical Team   *129*
You + Your Oncology Team = BFF   *132*
Chemo Time!   *135*
Soothing What Ails You   *139*
  Bone/Muscle Aches and Pains   *139*
  Constipation/Diarrhea   *145*
  Drowsiness/Insomnia   *146*
  Fatigue   *150*

Headaches   *152*
Numbness/Neuropathy   *154*
Nausea   *157*
Body Beautiful   *159*

Chapter 6. A Girl Thing   **161**

Hot Flashes   *165*
Infections   *166*
Bone Density/Osteoporosis   *167*
Sex   *169*
Eating Right/Staying Fit   *171*
   Be Prepared   *171*
   Eating Before Infusion   *172*
   Eating After Infusion   *174*
   Putting on the Pounds   *176*
   The Skinny on Weight Loss   *178*
   Changes to Taste   *178*
   The Rainbow Connection   *179*
   Nutritional Beauty   *181*

Chapter 7. The Integrative Approach   **183**

The Alternative Approach   *185*
   Accupuncture—A Point of Relief   *186*
   The Human Touch   *188*
   The Sound of Music   *193*
Finding Integrative Caregivers   *194*
Easing Dis-Ease   *197*

Chapter 8. Keeping the Faith   **203**

What to Do   *209*
Achieving Oneness   *213*
   Thy Will Be Done   *218*

Crisis = Opportunity *224*
A Family Affair *226*
Atlas in a Skirt *229*
But I'm Still Bald . . . *233*
The Quiet Hours *236*
The Prayer of Life *237*

Epilogue **243**

Parting Pearls *243*

Acknowledgments **257**

Index **261**

FOREWORD

Fashion Week is always high pressure; it's even more high pressure with a breast cancer diagnosis in the mix. I'm amazed I was able to do my cartwheels down the runway without anyone ever knowing I was in the middle of a crisis.

It was December of 1999 when I found out I had cancer. I did not share this news with anyone but my daughter, Lulu. Fearing what people would say, and just being too busy with Fashion Week coming up, I went for my lumpectomy and six weeks of radiation without whispering a word to anyone.

For thirty-five days at 7:00 A.M., I left my apartment way, way downtown and headed for my treatment way, way uptown. While this was happening, I was so busy concentrating on all I had to get done to get my collection ready that I didn't even think too much about how scary it all was. Luckily and amazingly, early detection worked its miracle. The lump I had was very small and was cleanly removed, and after I completed radiation, my prognosis was excellent.

It was all still unbelievable and overwhelming and frightening. When my doctors gave me the report that I was cancer free, the relief was incredible. I had faced one of the worst things that can happen to a woman, but I had also been spared something even more difficult: I did not have to go through chemo.

Many women aren't as blessed as I was. I've had some dear friends face the hair loss and the energy drain that chemotherapy creates; I find their spirit incredible. They understand the battle they must fight. But rather than let this get the better of them or try to pretend it's not happening at all, they embrace the life they have and do what they can to look like their usual selves while concentrating on getting better.

It's so obvious to me that the way a woman looks while she's going through chemo is going to affect the way she feels. I've seen it with my friends. One was just so amazing. She said, "Ok, I'm going to get through this, and make the best of it along the way," so she got the wig, the stencils, and the soft comfortable clothes, and with everything she went through, she really did look great.

I think a woman's true beauty is in her spirit, and there is no need to lie or camouflage what is happening to you. I believe the best thing any woman facing cancer and chemo can do is figure out what will make your spirit happy and do what you can to have that happen. Whatever colors appeal to you, whatever fabrics make you comfortable in your own skin, whatever type of wig or scarf or makeup lets you feel good about yourself—you owe that to yourself during this tough time.

Now, if you're someone with an in-depth knowledge of skin care or makeup or nutrition, you may already know some of the things Marybeth and Debbie will tell you inside this book. Most readers will appreciate how these two ladies have uncovered great information for their sisters in need, trying to help them feel better both inside and out while facing a very tough time. These authors have spoken to experts in so many areas where you may find yourself with a question or problem. They haven't limited themselves to appearance but also learned about things you can do with food and breathing and massage techniques to ease the side effects of chemo and make you feel relaxed and comfortable.

I love that they have created a space where a woman can find answers if something about her face or her body is suffering under a course of treatment she cannot refuse to endure: something that explains what's happening, and how to deal with it until it's over.

Women deserve to look in the mirror and feel uplifted and positive, and I think the best way to make that happen when you've got to have chemo is to commit to giving yourself all the comfort and kindness you can manage. Treat yourself to whatever you want, whatever works for you. Whether it's having a massage, taking a nap, talking to your friends, or participating in a group, make that your top priority and trust that everything else will fall into place.

I believe that if you stick with your nearest and dearest and concentrate your energy where you need it most, you will come out of this as I did, turning cartwheels and giving thanks for all the love and support people will show you. Let that wonderful energy in, and let it be part of your glow.

—Betsey Johnson
New York, NY

beauty
pearls

for
chemo
girls

Prologue

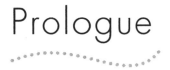

Our Panel of Experts

Anastasia of Beverly Hills—Anastasia Soare is recognized as a top beauty maven with a large and loyal celebrity clientele including Madonna, Jennifer Lopez, Oprah Winfrey, Penelope Cruz, and Sharon Stone.

Leah Berkowitz—New York–based fashion stylist Leah Berkowitz has dressed some of the most celebrated women in the world. Her work has appeared in most major fashion magazines including *Glamour, Seventeen, Lucky, Latina,* and *Io Donna,* as well as national advertising campaigns for companies including Cover Girl, Target, Verizon, and Oil of Olay.

Eivind Bjerke—With a reputation as the go-to stylist for "power heads" in Washington, DC, including Sandra Day O'Connor, Nancy Pelosi, and Hillary Clinton, Eivind is renowned for his exceptional style, premium service, and innovative solutions to any hair-related problem.

Oscar Blandi—One of the most respected and requested celebrity hair stylists working today, Oscar has created personalized looks for many of Hollywood's A-list actresses; his work and products are mainstays of top fashion and beauty bibles and his mission is to make gorgeous, salon-worthy hair attainable to all.

Amy Bragagnini, M.S., R.D.—Amy is a registered dietitian with a master's degree in nutrition and dietetics. She works at the Lacks Cancer Center, a state-of-the-art, environmentally advanced healing facility in Grand Rapids, Michigan, offering comprehensive inpatient and outpatient services and an integrative mind/body/spirit approach to treatment.

Michele Burke—Michele is the six-time nominated, two-time Academy Award–winning makeup artist sought out by filmmakers worldwide as one of the most versatile talents working in movies today.

Dr. Sandy Canzone—Dr. Canzone is a veteran doctor of Oriental medicine and a practitioner of Ayurvedic medicine who designed the St. Vincent Regional Cancer Centers, Full Spectrum Wellness Awakening to Life series for oncology patients in Santa Fe, New Mexico. She also practices homeopathy with extensive training in the Eastern understanding of nutrition.

Thomas A. Caputo, M.D.—Dr. Caputo is chief of Gynecological Oncology and Obstetrics and Gynecology at New York-Presbyterian Hospital.

Cheryl Chapman, R.N., L.M.T.—a pioneer in massage for cancer and mastectomy, Cheryl became a registered nurse in 1965 and was certified in massage in 1988. She studied Chinese medicine and massage in New York and China and in 1999 became Holistic Nurse Certified (HNC). Approved as a continuing education provider by the National Certified Board for Therapeutic Massage and Bodywork since 1992, Cheryl began teaching continuing education classes at national conferences, conventions, and massage schools throughout the United States. She also consults with massage schools, organizations, and spas. She is the author of *The Happy Breast Book*, a woman's guide to keeping her breasts healthy and happy.

Christine DeAngelo—Counting Kathlin Argiro, Polo Ralph Lauren, Chado Ralph Rucci, Pilar Rossi, and Jones Apparel Group among her clients, FIT graduate Christine DeAngelo is head designer for Flip Dresses, described as the "must-have trend setters" by *Women's Wear Daily*, *CosmoGirl!*, and *Seventeen* magazine.

Francine DeMarco—Graduated from FIT with a specialization in foundation garments, Francine is a fashion designer and stylist who has created designs for national ready-to-wear companies including Danskin, Disney, Warner Brothers, Limited Express, and Everlast. A former vice president of design for Tahiti Apparel, Francine is also cover stylist and beauty editor at *Prime Woman* magazine.

Louis Philippe DeMontpensier—Discovered by Halston and trained by Yves Saint Laurent, Louis Philippe was the makeup artist Jacqueline Kennedy Onassis depended on to keep her looking her best as she waged her own cancer battle.

Krista Dibsie—Krista is a licensed aesthetician, skin analyst, and entrepreneur. As the owner/developer of Skin Science, she has taken the concept of skin care to a new level, providing clients the opportunity to improve their skin's structure and function with an innovative line of products and services designed to perpetuate a beautiful, healthy complexion.

Rick DiCecca—This premier makeup artist has built a reputation for creating inspiring new looks each year based on the seasonal Estée Lauder color palettes. Regularly working with some of the world's most famous faces, Rick's innovative ideas and skilled artistry have established him as leader in the beauty and fashion business.

Dr. Lloyd Gayle—Chief of Plastic Surgery at New York–Presbyterian Hospitals, Doctor Gayle is also associate professor of clinical surgery and director of plastic surgery resident education at Weill Medical College of Cornell University.

Deann Geary—As founder of Tiffany Wigs, Deann has spent more than forty years working to provide custom-fitted wigs to chemotherapy patients worldwide and has developed a national reputation as one of the best wig salons for individuals afflicted with hair loss.

Harvey Gedeon—Estée Lauder Companies' executive vice president, global research and development, Harvey Gedeon is a world leader in the conceptualization and technical achievement of innovative beauty products.

Amy Gibson—Afflicted with alopecia at 13 years old and suffering complete hair loss by the time she was 30, soap opera and television star Amy Gibson developed her own wig line, featuring unique designs, material, and hair that combine style, comfort, and security. Amy's intention behind everything she does centers on "helping women feel and look complete from the inside out—from feeling like a victim to being victorious."

Dr. Noah Gilson—Dr. Gilson is a neurologist, professor of neurology, media liaison, and guest lecturer who is dedicated to the practice of neurosciences and the education of both medical students and the community at large regarding the complex nature of neurological topics.

Betsey Johnson—Award-winning fashion designer and breast cancer survivor is known around the world for her feminine and whimsical designs. Betsey opened her first boutique in 1969, and today oversees a retail empire that includes forty-five boutiques in the United States, Canada, and Britain, generating about $50 million in annual revenues.

Sheikh Abdur Rahman Kahn—Sheikh Rahman is a graduate of Islamic University Madinah and on the faculty of Shari'ah specializing in Islamic inheritance. He was principal of the Guyana Islamic Institute for eight years; Imaan at Windsor Forest West Masjid, Guyana; Imaan and head of Islamic Studies at the Muslim Community Center of Greater Rockford, Illinois; and is currently resident scholar and Khateeb at the Islamic Foundation in Chicago.

Dr. Ahmed Nezar Kobeisy—Dr. Kobeisy is a nationally recognized Muslim scholar, counselor, and religious leader. He is the director and resident scholar at the Islamic Learning Foundation who serves on the faculties at Le Moyne College (Syracuse, New York), Hartford Seminary (Hartford, Connecticut), and Syracuse University. He has also taught at the State University of New York at Oswego and Albany. Dr. Kobeisy served as the director and Imam of Islamic Centers in New York State for more than twenty years and is currently the Islamic chaplain at Syracuse University and offers training of Imams for U.S. mosques.

Theresa Loupuchin—Theresa is a licensed cosmetologist, trained in advanced skin care and makeup at the International School of Esthetics in Paris, and is the national spokesperson for the Look Good Feel Better® Foundation. An original volunteer who helped roll out the program in 1989, Theresa has been providing corporate and individual training in image consulting, one-on-one appearance assessment, and color consultation for over twenty years.

Gayle MacDonald, M.S., L.M.T.—A national and international health educator, writer, and body worker, Gayle has supervised massage students at the oncology unit at Oregon Health and Science University since 1994. She is the author of *Medicine Hands, Massage Therapy for People with Cancer* and *Massage for the Hospital Patient and Medically Frail Client.*

Reverend Dr. Patricia S. Medley—A breast cancer survivor, Dr. Medley is pastor of Hope Lutheran Church in Freehold, New Jersey, has served as chairperson of Bioethics of the CentraState Medical Center and of the Freehold Area CROP Walk for Hunger, president of the Interfaith Freehold Clergy Association, and is an advocate for survivors of domestic violence, the homeless, and those who struggle with addictions, as well as an advocate and educator in the area of sexual abuse and prevention of sexual abuse of children and parishioners.

Robert Lee Morris—The legendary, award-winning jewelry designer is globally recognized as a pioneer in the world of fine jewelry and fashion who has created a body of work that illuminates the body and nourishes the soul in an effortless fusion of the spiritual and the sensual.

Dr. Howard Murad—Widely acknowledged as one of the country's foremost authorities on skin care, board-certified dermatologist Dr. Murad has devoted his life to the science of internal and external skin care.

John Nies—Drafted into the NFL by the Buffalo Bills in 1990, John founded the Power Center in Red Bank, New Jersey, in 2002, developing an approach to fitness that's rooted in ancient Eastern wisdom but incorporates the benefits of modern fitness advances. He is the author of *Chi-Force, Living the Seven Disciplines*, an insightful approach to helping people find inner peace and balance while fulfilling their full potential, and sits on the advisory board of the Beauty Foundation for Women's Cancer Care.

The Oncology Nurses at Princeton Medical Group—Six oncology nurses with over seventy-five years combined experience in treating chemotherapy patients.

Oribe—The only hairstylist to have an exhibit featured at the Metropolitan Museum of Art in New York City, Oribe is considered one of the most innovative hair stylists of our time, with a client list that includes Jennifer Lopez, Sophia Loren, Penelope Cruz, Cate Blanchett, and Renée Zellweger. He has styled over 1,000 magazine covers and thousands of editorial fashion and beauty stories for *Vogue, Elle, Bazaar, GQ, Allure, Cosmo*, and *Glamour*, and has worked with the world's most renowned fashion photographers including Richard Avedon, Steven Meisel, Irving Penn, Annie Liebowitz, Mario Testino, and Francesco Scavullo.

Father Daniel Peirano—A former officer in the Peruvian army, Father Peirano spent twelve years in the American military and climbed to the rank of Captain before heeding the call to his spiritual vocation and joining the Congregation of Jesus in Mary Seminary in Bogotá, Colombia. He was ordained as a Roman Catholic priest in the diocese of Trenton, New Jersey, in May 2004 and serves as a parish priest at Saint Mary of the Seas parish, Long Branch, New Jersey, Diocese of Trenton, New Jersey.

Rabbi Jonathan Roos—Rabbi Roos leads the Monmouth Reform Temple in Tinton Falls, New Jersey, and is a member of the Rabbinic Cabinet of United Jewish Federation, past officer of the Capital District Board of Rabbis, and a member of the Central Conference of American Rabbis.

Dr. Samuel Schneider—Dr. Schneider is a Princeton-based psychotherapist with a special practice dedicated to helping oncology patients deal with the psychological and emotional issues surrounding their diagnosis and treatment.

Kurt Spellmeyer—Kurt Spellmeyer has practiced Zen meditation for thirty-two years and since 1994 has been director of the Cold Mountain Sangha at Rutgers University in New Jersey, where he is also an English professor. He has trained with Takabayashi Genki and Kangan Glenn Webb, founders of the Seattle Zen Center. In 1985, Spellmeyer completed his training under Webb Roshi and was authorized to teach. He received the dharma name Kankan Sensei (Ch. Guan Han, "Sees the Cold"), at a private ceremony with Webb in 1991.

Dr. Peter Staats—An internationally known physician, author, researcher, and lecturer on the subject of developing and implementing minimally invasive procedures for chronic pain, Dr. Staats is a fellow of the World Institute of Pain and the North American Neuromodulation Society and serves on the board of directors of the American Academy of Pain Medicine and the National Pain Foundation. His work has been highlighted on *Good Morning America, CBS Evening News,* and CNN.

Dr. Brian Torpey—A board-certified, fellowship-trained orthopedic surgeon, Dr. Torpey specializes in the treatment of conditions of the shoulder, knee, hip, sports medicine, shoulder and knee reconstruction, and orthopedic surgery.

Dr. Joann Weinrib—Chiropractor, nutritionist, and founder of New York City's Body Central, Dr. Weinrib has created an innovative, integrative center for healing in downtown Manhattan and the Hamptons, New York.

Dr. Patricia Wexler—A board-certified dermatologist specializing in dermatology and dermatologic surgery including state-of-the-art cosmetic surgical procedures, Dr. Wexler is one of the most sought after dermatologists in America and is recognized everywhere as an expert in the field of dermatology and dermatologic surgery.

Dr. Leonard Wright—Director of the Wege Institute for Mind, Body and Spirit at the Lack's Cancer Center in Grand Rapids, Michigan, Dr. Wright is a physician board certified in multiple medical subspecialties, including medical acupuncture. In 1989 he received a diagnosis of terminal brain cancer and applied a combination of Eastern and Western medical treatments to survive his disease and become a practitioner of, and advocate for, integrative medical cancer treatment therapies.

Survivors' Stories

Surviving cancer is a fantastic triumph. We've been there. We know.

From the moment of diagnosis until the day you put your wig away for good, life as you know it will change. Some of these changes may last forever—and most of them will be for the better. You'll be stronger. You'll know who your biggest supporters are. You'll understand your body and your mind in ways that prior to cancer might have been impossible. You won't sweat the small stuff. Every day, you'll find something to be happy about. It's inevitable. Facing this terrifying diagnosis, you'll come away from the experience with an insight unique to we who have been up the cancer mountain and made it safely to the other side.

We know this journey will be difficult. We understand the ups, downs, and radical shifts cancer treatment creates. Our hope is that by reading about our experiences, you will take our hearts and courage and join them with your own.

No one wants to feel alone during this challenging time. Believe that no matter where you are or what you are feeling, there is an enormous community of strength and support waiting to be called on. Take advantage of this support. Lean on those who want to help. Use our stories to inspire your own.

It is a great honor for us to share our experiences with you, our sisters in arms.

We salute you, chemo girls. We wish you every blessing as you make your way up the cancer mountain. We await your arrival on the other side.

Our Own Stories

Marybeth's Story

It wasn't being bald, or sick, or bloated that got to me. It was losing my eyelashes.

That's when I realized that I was actually pretty vain about my appearance and didn't want to spend the last three months of my chemotherapy treatments looking like an albino rabbit.

With no history of disease in my family, and possibly the smallest boobs on the planet to be afflicted with malignancies, I found a lump in my left breast one evening, discovered a smaller lump in the right one the next day, and within two weeks was deep in the world of surgery and illness, cancer, and chemotherapy.

As a writer and former television news producer, I delved into the research on my affliction with almost fundamentalist zeal. I wanted to know what had happened to me and what I could do to make sure it didn't happen again. I spent days trolling the Internet, reading every breast cancer hit my Google searches returned, trying to understand, trying to cope, trying to gain some sort of control over a body that in forty-three years had never once let me down but was now sporting a pair of weapons of mass destruction too small to fill a modest A-cup bra, yet deadly enough to kill me if I didn't act fast.

Luckily, I caught my disease early. I had my breasts removed, went deep into the chemo trenches, had reconstructive surgery, and am now doing fine. But while I was facing cancer down, the hardest thing for me to deal with was my image in the mirror. Sure, I was a fighter. I was determined to do whatever it took to make sure this cellular error didn't leave my husband a widower and my children motherless. And I knew, intellectually at least, that what I looked like was the least of my problems.

But it hurts to be bald. It's painful when eyebrows disappear, tongues swell, and the fringe of lashes a girl has taken for granted since babyhood lie like feathery memories on a pillowcase. It's tough to get up in the morning, and instead of seeing the face you've known your whole life, greet in the mirror a person who is supposed to be you, yet looks like a stranger.

I knew my insides were under attack. I knew that the chemo that was so difficult to endure was going to make sure I won the cancer war. But I didn't want to look like a sick person. I wanted to look like myself.

That's what brought me to the bookstores. Looking for all the inside tips and tricks other women who'd been down this road had already discovered, I found there was nothing on the shelves to help me—no books to explain what these necessary drugs would do to my hair and skin and energy— no guides to map out what I should expect during six months of treatment.

Debbie and I teamed up to do the work, and the result is this book.

Every woman facing disease deserves to understand what is happening when potentially lethal drugs are pumped into her medical port. She should be able to keep her skin, eyes, teeth, hair, hands, feet, mind, and spirit as healthy and vibrant as sickness will allow.

She shouldn't feel lost or hopeless. She should feel that in all the ways that matter, she's still in control.

If knowledge is power, think of these pages as a command post in your battle against disease. Learn about the drugs your doctor has prescribed, how they will affect your body, your mind, your metabolism, and your soul. Embrace this opportunity to face cancer down, and keep it between your psyche and your skin.

After years on the front lines of illness, I know this: all women are survivors. We're all beautiful. We deserve to look our best, no matter what the circumstances. So here's to chemo doing the dirty work inside, and here's to us, facing it down by putting our best foot (and skin and attitude) forward.

Good luck!

Debbie's Story

I learned at an early age that when someone is sick, someone else also suffers—usually in silence.

I was 24, my boyfriend was 28 when a blood clot formed in his leg and landed him in the hospital. His stay was short, but his recovery slow. Being young and impatient, I just wanted him to get better so we could get on with our lives.

Two years later, we were married and tried to put the illness behind us. But a year later, he was hospitalized for three weeks with deep vein thrombosis. This time, recovery was nine months.

Three years after that—just five weeks after I had given birth to our first child—a clot passed through his lung, but we continued to do our best to be a normal growing family. I delivered our second daughter, he went to work, and I continued to grow in my career as a cosmetics executive.

Then a virus attacked his pericardium. His heart stopped twice. The nurse told me to bring our two- and three-year-old girls to the Critical Care Unit to see him, and being something of an expert at hospital procedure by now, I knew that meant they thought he may die.

Luckily for us, his cardiologist came to the rescue, transferred him to a New York City hospital, and four weeks later, he was released to my care. He was 37. I was 33. Now, over a decade later, he continues to take many medications, mostly preventive, and goes to a hospital as a patient about every three years for something related—yet unrelated—to an illness that has no name.

I don't know if anyone who hasn't been a partner to a devastatingly ill person can understand the fear, the worry, the anger, and the exhaustion that dealing with disease brings. I was terrified at what could happen and furious at the dagger forever pointed at my family's happiness; yet, for the most part, I couldn't express any of these emotions for fear of how they'd affect my husband, our kids, our families—and myself.

Every day I work hard, stay strong, and try to ignore the pain this sickness in our lives triggers inside of me. But sometimes, the pressure leaks out. When my cousin was diagnosed with ovarian cancer and my college roommate found out she had breast cancer I experienced a sense of unease, unsure how I could help them when I was giving everything I had to my family.

In desperation, I reached out to a friend with HIV for advice. He had a lot of experience nursing dying friends, and he told me that the best way to cope with illness was to accept that it was happening, face it with all the courage I could muster, and stay positive.

This can be easier said than done. Depression and fear can paralyze even the closest, most well-intentioned friends. That's why I'm so happy to be writing this book. I wish I'd had it when I went to see my cousin and my college roommate so that I could share with them all the ways they could continue to look and feel good as they waged war against their disease.

I wish I could carry it with me so that if I receive the awful news that yet another person I know is facing one of life's biggest hurdles, I can present her with this handbook of hope.

I've been working in the beauty business for over twenty years, and there's one thing I know: a bit of confidence, a touch of beauty, and a sense of personal well-being can bring out the best in any woman.

Looking good is a huge step in the psychological battle to be well. It not only helps you but gives a sense of relief and hope to those who love you and want with all their hearts for you to look and feel as best you can.

The road ahead is tough, but I'm confident that the insight provided by the friends you'll meet inside this book will help you cope—and triumph—as you continue your journey to wellness.

The Survivors' Stories

Chris's Story

Late on a Saturday afternoon in January 2001, during an out-of-state visit with my mother, what felt like a bladder infection brought me to a local walk-in clinic. The staff doctor examined me and gave me a prescription to fix the problem. When that didn't do anything to help me, I knew "something" was wrong.

That something turned out to be ovarian cancer.

The news that I had this disease stunned me. I was 51, and as far as I knew, perfectly healthy. But I soon learned that the symptoms of ovarian cancer "whisper" to its victims, who can easily explain them away: occasional lower backaches, fatigue. Who doesn't have those once in a while? Sometimes I was exhausted, but I work hard and play hard, so that didn't strike me as strange. I felt bloated, but I'd like to meet the woman who hasn't experienced that. And the unexplained fifteen pounds I'd put on made me regret the loss of my trim figure and flat abdomen, but I just figured encroaching menopause was to blame for the fact that, standing sideways, I looked four months pregnant, because I certainly had not changed my eating or exercise habits.

It turns out that all of these were warning signs of the invisible invader growing inside me. The bloating especially indicated something was amiss, though I had no idea that the gurgling, sloshing, gastric noises emanating from my torso were not indigestion or the flu but a complex malignant mass.

Once I returned from my mom's house, I went to see my gynecologist, who ran the tests that found a six-inch tumor—Stage 2, Grade C. I immediately underwent a complete hysterectomy. Three weeks later, chemotherapy began.

My treatment involved eight hours of infusion. It would begin at 9 A.M. and end at 5 P.M. There were six in all, each one three weeks apart, and the side effects were very rough.

I lost my hair, my lashes, my eyebrows—within two weeks of my first treatment, all were gone. I gained forty pounds from the steroids and lack of exercise and had a face full of pimples too.

But that was not nearly as hard as the poisonous way the treatment made me feel. Forty-eight hours after leaving the doctor's office, I would be in bed with what seemed like the worst case of the flu imaginable. Pain coursed through my body, especially my legs. I couldn't read, or think, or watch television; my brain was unable to focus on anything. And this would last for seven days.

Once that first week passed, I would start to feel better. The second week things improved even more, and by the third week, I was feeling okay, but then I would have to go back and begin the nightmare again.

None of this was easy. What motivated me more than anything was a driving desire to live. I remember sitting on my sofa and thinking about the odds of beating this. My doctor told me that with treatment I had a 90 percent chance of recovery. I focused all my energy on that 90 percent and refused to let negative, scary thoughts bring me down.

Positive thinking is essential when facing this disease. I believe it helped me get to my current state of remission. It's been over eight years since my diagnosis, and I think of myself as being a lucky woman. With the help, love, and support of family, loved ones, and friends, I managed to get through a very difficult time.

Today I have my hair and my body back, and my life as well. The changes to my skin and self-image that were so hard to accept are all gone. Sure, I'm a little heavier than I was before, but I feel great. More importantly, I take nothing for granted. I still go for regular follow-up appointments with my oncologist and have regularly scheduled cat scans and ultrasounds. Ovarian cancer symptoms may indeed whisper, but I'm paying close attention to the sound of my body, and I'm very proud and happy to report that the only noise coming from inside me is the happy song of survival.

May that song fill your heart and your life, in the days and years to come.

Laura's Story

"Get a mammogram. Now!"

The command came from my sister that Monday morning in May 1999. We were on the phone, and I was describing to her what felt like a pea-shaped lump in my breast when she stopped listening and told me to go get it checked.

We had reason to worry. My mom had died at a young age from ovarian cancer, and I had already had a breast fibroadenoma, which is a benign tumor commonly found in young women's breasts. Within twenty-four hours of our conversation, I was listening to the radiologist's comforting words that it was merely a cyst. When I recalled for him my mother's early diagnosis and fate, he became annoyed and told me that too many young women were "making mountains out of molehills." He told me to forget about the lump and come back in two years.

Livid, I marched out of his office, purchased copies of my films, and made an appointment with the chief breast surgeon at Memorial Sloan Kettering Cancer Center in Manhattan. Initially told that I would have to wait five months for an opening, I recounted my family history, and an appointment became available for the following week.

When my husband and I arrived at the doctor's office, a sea of women sat in the lobby, patiently waiting for their chance to see the surgeon. After three hours, my husband began to express his irritation, but I knew there was no way I was going to leave before I'd had my time with the doctor.

I did indeed have cancer. I had a lumpectomy, and after learning it was malignant, I went deep into research mode, calling doctors all over the country and trying to decide what course of treatment would give me the best chance of raising my three children to adulthood and growing old with my husband. A recommendation from a doctor at Dana Farber in Boston made the most sense to me. Two months after finding the lump, I underwent bilateral mastectomies and followed the surgeries with six months of chemotherapy.

Because my husband and I had lived through my mother's battle with cancer, we knew what we were facing. I sat down with my children and explained as best I could what was going to happen to me. I think the honesty helped. My eight-year-old son came up with a signal that meant he needed private time to ask me questions. Being open and direct with them seemed to help them cope with my illness better than I remembered being able to when my own mom was sick.

Chemotherapy was not easy, but I was determined to keep a positive attitude and never give in to cancer. I went to every treatment wearing my favorite loafers and a soft pashmina and carrying my designer bag. My clothes were my chemo armor. I also did my best to keep my sense of humor and never let anyone treat me like an invalid.

A week after my first treatment, our family went to Lake Placid, and I proved to everyone how strong I still was. I water-skied, hiked up White Face Mountain, and saw more beauty and felt more inner strength than I had ever before experienced. And while my doctors didn't love these antics, the constant activity and striving to be normal empowered me. I visualized myself as a warrior and kept my sights on victory.

Today, ten years have passed since my sister insisted I get to the doctor. I am healthy and happy and full of life. But I believe that the one downside to being ever upbeat and positive about my situation was that to this day no one realizes how difficult a journey it was for me, both physically and emotionally. I was so very scared, and tired, and worried about my family. Looking back, maybe it would have been better if every now and then I relaxed and let someone else hold up the world.

Over the years, I've come to see cancer as a gift: it has taught me to appreciate my life in a way I hadn't before. I cherish each day like stars sprinkled from heaven, and I value all the love that has been there for me.

I wish each of you this gift—the joy of the rest of your life.

Patricia's Story

My husband and I were making love just before Mother's Day in May 2004 when he discovered the lump in my right breast. The next day my friend, a breast surgeon, did an ultrasound. We looked at the screen, and as doctors, we couldn't deny the truth—I had cancer.

As a gynecologist, I knew what I had to do. First, I contacted the radiologist who had been following me for the

last seven years with annual digital mammographies and
ultrasound examinations to track the microcalcifications discovered on my baseline mammography back when I was 35,
and arranged a biopsy. Then I enlisted my best friend from
medical school, who is a breast oncologist, to find excellent
doctors not emotionally attached to me because of work,
school, or friendship, to be on my medical team.

Within two weeks, my lumpectomy was over, but the
pathology report was not great: a 2.6-cm hormone-receptive
positive, HER 2/neu tumor and 26 lymph nodes were
removed; two nodes were positive. I had extensive vascular
invasion, and one of the eight margins was borderline. Re-
excision didn't get me the clean margin I sought.

This was frustrating—scary too. My mother had been
diagnosed with breast cancer at 64, and I had thought my
digital mammography and ultrasound screenings, done each
year, six months apart, would protect me from advanced
disease. But it seems I have "camouflage breasts" that
essentially hid the mass. During my biopsy, the radiologist
admitted that had I not shown her the tumor by palpation
[touch], she would not have seen it on the ultrasound.

At 42, with a thriving medical practice, a happy marriage,
and a young child, my number-one priority was survival. I
chose aggressive chemotherapy, a mastectomy, and followed
that surgery with six weeks of daily radiation.

Without a doubt, chemotherapy was the most challenging
part of the journey. My hair fell out, my bones hurt, and
each treatment was harder than the one before.

Even more difficult was the fact that my husband had to
be away for six and a half weeks of my treatment. Though
this was rough, his absence taught me to lean on people.
Like many women, I had a hard time asking for help. But I
couldn't cook, and my daughter needed to eat, so friends

would come to my house and leave meals for us in a cooler
we had waiting on the back porch.

I continued to work throughout treatment, changing my
schedule to accommodate my needs. Finances were part
of the reason, but it was more a desire for normalcy that
motivated me; being busy and professionally engaged gave
me back that sense of control I'd lost after diagnosis.

I also made it a point to take care of myself, going for
regular facials and massage. A cosmetologist taught me
how to draw on my missing eyebrows. I drank lots of water,
exercised, and never went anywhere without my wig.

Cancer was a hard road for me. The bone pain took three
years to end. Because estrogen fed my cancer, my doctor
shut down my ovaries with Lupron, and that threw me into
early menopause. Between a slowing metabolism and all
the steroids given with the cancer-fighting drugs, I gained
25 pounds, and during one especially long airline flight I
developed lymphedema.

But for every problem, I found a solution. Tired of taking
hormone-suppressing medications, I stopped the Lupron
and had my ovaries laproscopically removed. I work out
almost every day to control my weight. Whenever I get on a
plane I wear a special sleeve and glove to compress my arm.
And though I really miss my breast, I decided against reconstruction because of a theory I'd heard that this could trigger
vascular growth and recurrence.

These changes to my body are very hard on my husband.
I know he looks at me and wonders where his sexy wife
went. But I am at peace with my decisions. I want to raise
my daughter. I want to grow old with my husband. I want
to be cancer free, and I will continue to do whatever it
takes to make these things happen. Extraneous issues don't
bother me anymore. Staying alive is what matters now.

I hope you are able to find a similar kind of peace within yourself, along with the strength to stand by your decisions, and the wisdom to do what you know is best for you.

Rosemarie's Story

"Could you feel this for me?" I asked my best friend that day back in 1997. I'd just gotten out of the shower at her house, and the ball I'd found in my left breast a few days earlier was still there, still hurting, still making me feel that the walls of my life were about to come crashing down.

I had reason to be nervous. I was only 27, but my mom had gone through breast cancer at 42, and I remembered all too well her battle to be well. It was probably the fear of it happening to me that made me ignore my breasts for the most part—not doing self-exams, not wanting to ever have to face that "what if . . . ?" moment.

But there I was, looking anxiously at my friend, who could feel the lump just under my armpit. She tried to reassure me, saying it was probably nothing, but suggested I call my doctor, just to be sure. So I got in touch with my mother's gynecologist, who was also mine, and knowing our family history, he insisted I come in right away. After examining me, he said it could be a cyst but wanted me to have a mammogram and then a sonogram. Within a day, confirmation of what I had secretly dreaded had come to pass: I had breast cancer.

Because of its size and location, I had a lumpectomy. The pathology report showed that the in situ tumor had been excised successfully, was hormone-receptor positive and HER 2 Negative, and there had been no spread.

This news was something of a double-edged sword; though these results were good, the next steps were not at all clear. I went to seven different oncologists and each one told me I could aggressively treat the cancer with radiation and chemotherapy—or forget the chemo and just do radiation. The choice was mine.

I look back on this now and wonder what these doctors were thinking, leaving such an enormous decision to a terrified twenty-seven-year-old without a clue as to what should be done. I had no one to advise me. My mother was wracked with guilt that she had done this to me, my sister and father were terrified that I was sick. I was really, really scared of what it would do to me after witnessing my mother's struggles with chemo.

I decided to have eight and a half weeks of radiation. When it ended, I felt fine and sort of relieved. It hadn't been that bad, and now it was over.

Three and a half years later, though, another lump appeared in my left armpit. I was instantly overwhelmed with fear, anger, and guilt. I couldn't believe it was happening again. I felt sure that had I chosen chemo before, I wouldn't be facing a second bout of cancer now.

My surgeon removed the new tumor and 27 lymph nodes from under my arm. This time around, there was no choice about treatment. Chemo was coming. The fight for my life had begun.

In a way, I was happy for the clear course of action. I was afraid, but at the same time it felt good to have a doctor take charge of this aspect of my life and give me direction on what I had to do.

I also received, in the midst of all this horror, an amazing gift. About three months earlier, I'd started dating a great guy. Once he learned I had cancer, I was sure he'd be gone. Instead of leaving me, however, he became my savior. Not baldness or nausea or scary moments of pain could make him leave my side. His strength centered me. Together, we made it through.

Today, six years after my last treatment and ten years after that fateful day at my best friend's house, I'm cancer free. I'm also married to my wonderful man, and we're hoping my doctor will soon give us the go-ahead to start a family. We know there's a chance I may not be able to have a baby, but we're ready to give it a try.

Cancer has taught me that yesterday is history and tomorrow a mystery. All we have is today. I suppose that's why it's called the present!

I wish all of you this gift: the wonder and joy of today.

CHAPTER 1

The Power of Makeup

Wearing makeup for the first time is a powerful experience.

Applying that first bit of lip gloss or mascara to her face, a young girl suddenly sees the beautiful possibilities of her life staring back at her from the mirror. Her eyes sparkle. Her lips shine. Her confidence soars.

Whether or not makeup is an important element in your daily life, few women will argue with its allure. Cosmetics highlight our best features and camouflage our perceived flaws. A bit of eyeliner, some well-applied blush, a bit of cream on the mouth, and voila! We take what we've been born with and make it better.

Makeup is fun. Who doesn't enjoy being fussed over in a department store by an aesthetician brushing powder over our cheeks? What woman wouldn't be thrilled to win one of those magazine makeover contests, where professionals take her skin and hair and clothing and create a whole new look?

For a majority of women, appearance is vitally important.

It projects to the world how we feel about ourselves. It creates the external shell through which our inner beauty radiates. Through our style in hair and clothing and makeup, we project an essential element of our personal power—the way we want to be seen.

Imagine how hard it is when the cancer strikes, the treatment begins, and the carefully cultivated look we've spent our lives developing suddenly disintegrates. Think of the difficulty losing your hair, or your eyelashes, or your shape would create in your life.

Go deeper. Picture yourself too nauseated to eat, too frightened to sleep, or too tired to get up. Imagine your skin breaking out, your clothes not fitting properly, and those people who care about you unable to retrieve what you've lost.

You may have always considered yourself a woman who could handle any crisis—but in the face of the internal and external emergency cancer creates, you may wonder where you'll find the strength to carry on.

Looking Good/Feeling Better

Years ago, women undergoing chemotherapy had to deal with the breakdown in their face and bodies without much sympathy. Doctors working to cure them of disease were not particularly interested in hearing how awful being bald made their patients feel. Few knew how to draw on missing eyebrows or where to go for a flattering wig. Women spent little time on the finer points of skin care. Nausea may leave a woman exhausted. Fear may make sleep impossible. But these issues were deemed trivial. Fighting for their lives, women were essentially told to forget about how they looked— and felt—and focus solely on their cancer.

Chemo girls did as they were told. They became warriors against their illness. Many prevailed, but few laughed during the process. Self-esteem took a nosedive. Depression was common. A positive attitude was not.

In the late 1980s, this scenario underwent a dramatic change. Medical professionals found that women who maintained a more normal appearance during chemotherapy had a much more positive outlook about their health situation. They responded better to treatment. They were less likely to be depressed and more inclined to view their care and future in an optimistic way.

These observations have sparked a revolution in women's cancer care. No longer rejecting the notion that looking good actually does make a girl feel better, doctors are partnering with hair stylists, aestheticians, psychologists, and holistic practitioners to educate their patients about what they can do to alleviate some of the physical and psychological hardships of chemotherapy.

Since 1989, The Look Good Feel Better Foundation® has spearheaded the effort to help women cope with the physical changes cancer brings. This not-for-profit organization partners with the American Cancer Society and the Personal Care Products Council to provide female cancer patients with the tools they need to make it through treatment looking as well as they can. Patients can attend these sessions in participating hospitals. Local hair, makeup, and skin care professionals volunteer their time and expertise to work with the facility's inpatients, teaching them how to make the most of what they've got.

National spokeswoman Theresa Loupuchin describes a class this way: "These women know what their problems are. It's all visible. The first thing I say is 'Ladies, we're going to have fun today. We're going to play with makeup. We're going to figure out what your specific beauty needs are, and we're going to address them. Because today, no one has cancer. We're just women looking for ways to take what we've got and make it better."

Like a balm on sore skin, relief flows from the participants.

"It happens at every class," Theresa says. "Women go from being closed like shutters to being open and sharing. There are no tears. There's lots of laughter. Wigs come off. People talk about their kids, their jobs, their favorite cleansers. Medicine and doctors and treatments are forgotten, because they're not patients anymore—they're women."

Chemo girls lucky enough to reap the rewards of a Look Good Feel Better session will attest to the wonders some training and advice can bring. The Foundation reaches about 50,000 patients per year.

In the United States alone, more than 650,000 women undergo cancer treatment every year. No single foundation can help them all. That's what this book is for—to give chemo girls all the information they need to look good and feel better throughout their cancer treatment, in the privacy of their own homes.

Why It Still Matters

No woman wants to experience unwanted, radical changes to her appearance. Regardless of how she views her hair or figure, if one of these features changes or disappears—she's going to mourn the loss.

Cancer has an impact on more than our outer shell. It strikes at the heart of our being. Once healthy and strong, we're now sick and scared. Where confidence ruled, confusion reigns. In the face of this physical assault, beauty becomes ever more illusive. A wig will cover baldness, but only faith and trust can soothe fear. Foundation may camouflage flaws, but only effective treatments will alleviate a rocky stomach, pounding headache, or aching bones.

True beauty is more than skin deep. It emanates from within, encompassing our bodies, spirits, and souls. It's the sum total of everything that we are. That's why we spent so much time speaking with professionals across the spectrum of personal care. Looking at all the appearance-affecting side effects chemotherapy can cause, we searched nationwide for experts to offer solutions for the internal and external problems chemo girls face. Every single professional quoted in these pages enthusiastically accepted our invitation to help women in need.

Utilize the pearls of wisdom these amazing people have provided. Spend a bit of time understanding their advice; then go on out and let the world see you as you are—a strong and confident person who is in control.

The essential truth we learned from our experts is, if looking good makes you feel better—then feeling good makes you look better. The concepts are intertwined. Take advantage of them. Care about your physical self, your emotional self, and your spiritual self. It's not only a way to retain normalcy during sickness, but it's a chance to show the world—and yourself—that you're the same feminine, wonderful person you've always been.

Refusing to give into illness is an act of hope and courage we hope you'll engage in whenever you're feeling up to the task. Focus on your needs, be proud of who you are, and remember that when this is over, you'll come out of the experience stronger and better than you ever were before.

Cancer is a temporary setback. Let it run its course without losing your dignity, your self-respect, or your confidence. Keep your head high, your heart calm, and your eyes on the prize. You will be more than fine. You will be fabulous.

CHAPTER 2

The Mane Event

THE SURVIVORS REMEMBER

Marybeth: I never loved my curly hair, so when I learned it was all going to fall out, I selected a poker-straight wig. It was my dream hair, and that made dealing with baldness much easier. Then, when my curls grew back, they were softer and finer. Now I think of chemo as a cure for coarse curls!

Chris: I was blow-drying my hair when fistfuls started flying all over the bathroom. I tried to vacuum my head with a hand vacuum, but that didn't work, so my friend shaved it for me. While my wig was lovely, I never really got used to it. Then the World Trade Center towers collapsed. Somehow my hair just really didn't matter much anymore. On September 12, 2001, I put the wig away.

Laura: I was lucky (or perhaps unlucky) enough to have gone through a "Cancer Training Program" via my mother's ovarian cancer and learned quickly that losing your hair is more traumatic if it happens slowly. So I cut my hair very short and then shaved my head when the hair first began to fall out.

Patricia: As a doctor, I thought it was important not to alarm my patients, so I didn't go anywhere without my wig. The only time I went without a head cover was at home, and a lot of my male colleagues never knew I'd lost all my hair. After treatment ended, I went to Jamaica for five days and used that time to get out of the habit of wearing a wig and get comfortable having very short hair.

Rosemarie: Losing my hair was the hardest part of chemo for me. It was long and dark and a big part of my self-image. My mom took me out for my wig, which looked exactly like my real hair. It became my security, and when the days grew too hot to wear the wig, I went out and bought lots of different-colored bandanas. It was of fun, in a making-the-best-of-it kind of way.

The Side Effects
hair thinning/total hair loss

The Pearls

Once the shock of a cancer diagnosis wears off, fear of baldness usually sets in. Hope and disbelief commingle. Our hair, after all, is such an essential part of our self-image. No woman wants to believe hers will fall out. No one wants to imagine herself bald.

"There's a lot of unreality when people are told they're going to experience hair loss," says Deann Geary, founder and owner of Tiffany Wigs. "They don't really want to think about what they'll look like without hair, or think about how, when it's growing back, their hair will be very short."

Amy Gibson agrees. "Hair is such an important part of us. Most women are taught that it's our crowning glory, our mane, our sensuality, our sexuality."

But Amy, who lost all her hair to alopecia at 30 years old and developed her own wig line featuring unique designs, material, and hair that combine style, comfort, and security, says the key to dealing with its loss is always to remember that femininity is in our essence, not our tresses.

"Remember, girls," she tells us, "we're more than our hair."

What's Going On

Because cancer cells reproduce rapidly, chemotherapy is specifically formulated to kill any cells that behave in that quickly multiplying way. That's why our hair is affected; the drugs we take to kill cancer can't differentiate between a fast-growing tumor cell and a healthy hair cell, so they attack both. While that's great for our future health, it can be devastating to our present self-esteem.

If your treatment side effects include losing your hair, nothing you do will stop it from falling out. Tight bands and cold caps, once thought to reduce blood flow to the hair follicles and limit chemotherapy exposure, have proven to be ineffective. Rather than pretend it won't happen, or let the fear of baldness get the better of you, the best advice we can provide for coping with this very visible side effect is to be prepared.

"A friend of mine was facing chemo," remembers Estée Lauder's premier makeup artist Rick Dicecca. "I was trying to prepare her by going over the side effects. As soon as I mentioned cutting off a clump of her hair so we could match it to a wig, she said, 'Maybe I won't lose my hair.' I knew she was just not dealing with the reality of what was going to happen, so I told her, 'Honey, you're going to look like Tweety Bird a week after treatment starts, so let's get busy.'"

Rick says the first order of business for all chemo girls must be to get the facts regarding your treatment so that you know what to expect. "If you're going to lose your hair, don't sit around waiting to look bad, and don't be afraid to look good. There's a lot you can do to get ready before the first hair falls out."

First Things First—Buy a Wig

All our experts agree: once told you're going to lose your hair, your first order of business should be finding a wig. "The minute you're told you're getting chemo, start shopping," Amy advises, "or at least get yourself familiar with what's out there."

Deann adds that it's best to buy your wig while still sporting your own tresses. "Sometimes people want to be different, but most times people want to look like themselves. It's easier to do that if we see them with their natural hair."

Oribe, considered one of the most innovative hair stylists of our time, agrees. "My clients have the best experience when they come to me before the chemo starts. That way, I can see their hair and match the color, the wave form, the style." He adds the key reason to move quickly:

"It gives a woman a nice feeling of security to know she has a wig that looks great and is waiting, ready to be worn as soon as she needs it."

You can purchase wigs online, from a salon, or through a community wig bank. The trick to making the best, most comfortable choice is to give yourself enough time to find what you want in style, color, material, and price.

"Bring a friend with you," Deann says. "Someone whose judgment you trust. Don't try to copy your own hair exactly, but make a selection based on what looks natural and what will be easy to maintain. You're already going through enough; you don't need the added work of a difficult hairstyle."

Being comfortable in your hairpiece is essential. This means a secure fit, a comfortable cap, and a style that brings out the best in your face.

"The patient needs to consider style and comfort together," Oribe says. "Many women don't want people looking at them because they're bald. A wig is something that will make it more comfortable for you to go out; you've covered your head and you look attractive."

Washington, DC, hair stylist Eivind Bjerke agrees. "Your hair is the frame of your face, and when chemo causes it to fall out, it's as if your frame has been broken. But if you put a beautiful wig on, one that makes you look good, even if you are not feeling your best, you can still look your best."

Choosing a Wig

Oscar Blandi, whose clients include many of Hollywood's A-list actresses, recommends being open to having fun when choosing a wig. "I help my clients pick out a wig that best represents their personality and resembles their hair's characteristics," he says. "I tell them to play with different colors, and it can become very invigorating because you have so many colors and textures with wigs that would not necessarily work with your own hair."

All our experts emphasize the opportunity this crisis can represent: a chance to break away from your old look and create an amazing new change.

"I try to turn all of this into an opportunity," Amy says. "I often ask my clients, do you, or did you, like your hair? And most say no, or it could be better, and I tell them, here's your chance to look any way you want."

"My first question is to ask if they're pleased with their look," Eivind says. "If your hair is going to fall out, that's pretty traumatic. Some people decide now is the time to try a look they've never had before. In a situation like this, there are a lot of choices available."

"With so many inexpensive, synthetic wigs to choose from, you can be a redhead one day, and a brown bob the next," Oribe says. "Though it's a lot to ask during this time, I think having a sense of humor can be very important."

All our hair experts have stories of women who decided that baldness gave them the green light to be outlandish, including Eivind, who remembers that "one woman came to me with whatever hair she had left and told me to give her a Mohawk. So I did. And she was gorgeous."

Oribe maintains that the quandary chemotherapy creates with our hair can also present the possibility of breaking out of yourself, if you are willing to give something new a try. "Consider this your chance to have fun with your look," he says. "Live out a fantasy. Be a diva."

Synthetic or Human—Let's See What's Best

Wigs are made of either human hair or synthetic fiber. While it might seem that human hair wigs would be the preference, every expert we asked said that for chemotherapy patients, synthetic was the better way to go.

"Synthetic is less bulky," Deann explains. "The strands are thinner and it actually looks more like human hair than human hair does. The curl and style stay in, so you wash it, dry it overnight, and wear it the next morning."

"Human hair wigs require greater maintenance," she continues, "more washing, more styling. They react to the weather, so in the rain the curls come out and they generally cost around ten times more than a synthetic."

"They can look great," Oribe says about human hair wigs, "but they're very expensive and the maintenance is harder. A hairdresser has to blow it out for you, unless you are very crafty, and when you're not feeling great, who wants to blow out a wig?"

Synthetic wig prices run from the $50 range for an off-the-shelf, coarse fiber wig to nearly $1,000 for a custom synthetic made with soft, human-hair-like fibers. Human hair wigs are usually custom made and prices run around $3,500 or higher.

"Generally, human hair is for teenagers," Deann observes. "They really want to have the hair, and they don't seem to mind the time it takes to wash and maintain it."

She sums up the general wisdom from our experts, saying, "For chemotherapy patients, ease is the most important thing. You don't want your wig care to become an ordeal. And from that perspective, the benefits of synthetic are obvious."

Insurance

Many insurance companies will pay for a wig or reimburse you up to a certain amount toward your wig purchase, as long as you provide them with a prescription from your doctor that reads "cranial prosthesis."

Find out what your coverage will allow, and let that figure help inform any choice you make about how much you want to spend on your wig. It is also a good idea to find out exactly what type of information your carrier will want to see on the purchase invoice so that you are able to submit the correct paperwork.

We didn't find any stores willing to deal directly with their client's insurance companies, but all of them provide invoices to send in with the claim for reimbursement.

"You want an insurance invoice that fits the requirements of the carrier, with diagnosis and procedure codes,"

Deann explains. "To the best of my knowledge, no government insurance covers wigs, but there are some wonderful companies that cover the price of the piece and the services. Others drive you crazy. I do my best with whatever help is necessary to facilitate payment."

When making your wig purchase, be sure to inquire as to the paperwork the manufacturer or salon will generate on your behalf, and ask if they will support you by making a phone call or providing additional information should your carrier make that request.

Comfort + Style = Your Best Choice in Caps, Color, and Cut

Caps

Though people see the color, material, and style of the wig, it is the cap underneath and the amount of fiber or hair on top that separates the comfortable wig from one that is, frankly, unwearable.

Amy recommends a cap made from a gauze-like, nearly transparent material called a monofilament.

"Perspiration can cause sores and rashes," she explains. "People think they're having an allergic reaction to the wig, but they're not—they've just got a wig that is too heavy. Your scalp has to be able to breathe.

"Here's the rule," she says. "Hold the wig up to the light and look at it from the inside. If you can't see through it, you can't breathe through it, and it won't be comfortable. Choose a different cap."

Handmade caps are constructed from light material with the strands of hair sewn individually into the cap. Machine-made caps have rows of hair sewn into ribbons, making them a little bit heavier.

"Some people are so sensitive, they have to have a hand-made cap," Deann says. "For others, a machine-made one works fine. It's like the princess and the pea. Only you can know which cap is right for you, and you'll know as soon as you put it on."

A wig wearer herself, Deann knows that no matter how good the wig looks, "If it's not comfortable on a person's head, it's going to be an ordeal to wear." She devised a series of measurements and redesigns every cap to custom fit her client's head. "The fit is hugely important," she says. "Since this is a blind item and people generally don't know what it's supposed to feel like, we're always making changes and adjustments."

Many wigs have Velcro tabs that allow the wearer to adjust the bands for a better, noncustom fit. Amy's wigs also feature scarf and eyeglass loops to make accessorizing and living in your wigs more convenient.

Deann advises searching for the wig that feels right from both a fit and style perspective. "The difference is personal. It's not so much handmade versus machine-made cap, but what does it feel like? What do you look like?"

Oribe seconds that opinion. "It's almost like buying a shoe. The fit and the style have to be right, and you can't really know until you put it on."

Color

The color of your wig is an entirely personal choice. While most people stick with their natural shade, some brunettes go blond or auburn while blondes may choose jet black. There is no right or wrong decision; it's all about what makes you look good and feel at home in your wig.

"You need to feel comfortable with the way you look," Eivind says.

Amy agrees. "It's not just how you look; it's about living in this foreign thing that has to become innate. That's the challenge, not covering something up but making the wig a part of you, as real as possible, that makes the difference.

"Take the wig into natural sunlight," she advises. "Go outside or to a window and study the color. Do not make your color choice by looking at the wig in fluorescent light or lamplight, as any light other than natural will give off a different hue and not necessarily be correct."

When considering shades, watch how different colors affect the look of your face. "Most women are off with their hue by about a half step," Amy says. "I would say about 90 percent of the time, I hold out another color, close but just a little richer, a little bit different, and they see it right away how their lips pop, their eyes pop. Suddenly they are able to see their beautiful features."

"You can use the wig to play up your other features," Oscar says. "Beauty doesn't disappear just because your hair does."

Cut

If your natural hair is long, Deann recommends getting a shorter haircut. Select a shorter-styled wig to ease the transition once treatment ends and your hair begins to grow back.

"You're not going to want to wear the wig that much once your own hair starts to come in," she says. "Think about shorter hair. When your hair begins to grow, you can transition from the wig in a much faster way."

"Shorter wigs are also easier to maintain," she says. "Longer fibers tend to get matted and natty over time."

Eivind agrees. "If you pick a long wig, you'll need more than one because the washing and drying take longer. You'll need a professional to help correct problems that arise over time, which means leaving it at a salon."

Amy has designed wigs that women can wear swimming or during intimacy. She believes lifestyle should inform the type of wig you select. "Are you active? Are you going to be dating? Consider these questions when choosing. It's important that you still live your life during treatment. Are you a couch potato? You don't want to be couched out in a $2,000 wig. It's better to get something less expensive. Give it a great cut that flatters your face and accommodates the life you'll continue to live throughout your treatment."

Oribe advises chemo girls to select a wig with bangs "because bangs hide the hairline, and without them, the look screams 'wig.'" He says a bob is a great choice because bangs work well with the style. They also help camouflage missing eyebrows, and take some attention away from thinning or lost eyelashes.

Wigs generally have more hair than a person's head, which can add to the heat and discomfort. Many wig salons will customize a client's choice, shaping and styling the piece so that it is lighter and easier to wear. You can bring a wig you have purchased to your hairdresser, put it on, and have it cut and styled as if it were your natural mane.

"The minute a lady puts the wig on, I forget that it's a wig and cut it as if it's her hair," says Oribe. "I thin it out where it's too heavy and work with her to continue the illusion that it's real hair."

Regardless of your wig's cut, Deann wants you to remember: "You don't want to be in a wig any longer than you have to, especially when you were thrown into it through circumstances that you would not have chosen on your own. So when you make your selection, keep in mind that this is only a short-term accessory, and choose the wig that you feel will be easiest to transition away from, once your treatment is over."

Measuring for a Custom Wig

Here is how Deann measures for a Tiffany custom wig:

Before you start: Pin hair as flat and as tight as possible before taking the measurements. This will eliminate bulges that distort head contours.

1. **The circumference of the head:** Measure all around the head. Position the tape measure so its edge follows the hairline around the head and the nape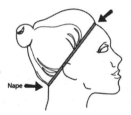

of the neck. (Average measurement is 22 inches.)

2. From the forehead to nape of the neck: Measure from the hairline at the center of the forehead straight back over the crown to the center of the hairline at the nape of the neck. (Average measurement is 13½ inches.)

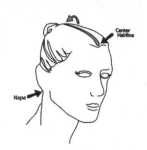

3. Ear to ear across the front hairline: At front of ear, measure from the hairline at base of sideburn, up across the hairline along the forehead to the same point in front of the other ear. (Average measurement is 11½ inches.)

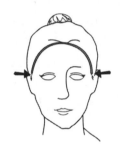

4. From ear to ear over the top of the head: Measure from the hairline directly above the ear across the top of the head to the hairline directly above the other ear. (Average measurement is 11 inches.)

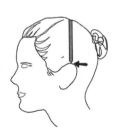

5. Point to point: From temple to temple across the back of the head. (Average measurement is 14 inches.)

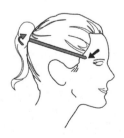

6. Nape of the neck: Measure the width of the hairline across the nape of the neck. (Average measurement is 6 inches.)

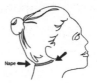

When the Wig Won't Work

You have kids who don't like to see you bald, but you've had enough of the cap for one day. You're relaxing at home when the doorbell rings. You're lying in bed and your head is cold. It's hot and you just don't feel like putting on your wig.

There'll be many times during your chemotherapy experience when your wig won't work. That's when you'll want some scarves or turbans to wear around the house, out to the store or dinner, or to pop on your head should the FedEx guy unexpectedly show up at the front door.

Turbans in cotton or velour are essential during treatment. They're wash-and-wear alternatives to your wig that will keep your head comfortable and cool if you're lounging around the house and warm while you're asleep.

"I wear velour turbans because my head gets really cold. If that doesn't happen to you, cotton is fine," says Amy. "I also have scarves that I wear alone or to accessorize my wig."

Oribe is a big fan of scarves. "There are different ways to wrap your head. You can look in fashion magazines for ideas or follow the celebrities. Jennifer Lopez looks great wearing scarves that cover her entire head. It's a lot more comfortable than wearing a wig."

Theresa Lopuchin suggests coordinating your scarf with

the rest of your outfit. "This is not a fun time, but you have to figure out how to have fun with it," she says. "I love the patterned scarves; you can pick colors that bring out your facial features and do your best to feel fabulous."

Scarf-Tying Options

The Basics

1. Fold a large square, 32"–36" diagonally, and drape it low over the forehead. Then, bring the ends to the back.
2. Finish by (using any of steps 2–4) looping (tie ends in a bow over point).
3. Finish by bundling (knot ends and fold point around bundled ends; secure point inside band).
4. Finish by coiling (cross ends over point and coil to front; intertwine coils for a continuous band and fold back, point up, inside crossed area). If a scarf is too small to accomplish scarf tying, fold it off center to make a larger cap. If the ends are short, band with a second scarf and finish with a decorative tie.

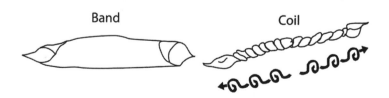

Band   Coil

Band and Coil Options

5. Band (fold opposite corners of a square to center, overlapping points, and fold again to desired width).

6. Coil (twist a band from the center out for an even coil). Several simple, decorative head wraps may be created using bands and coils.

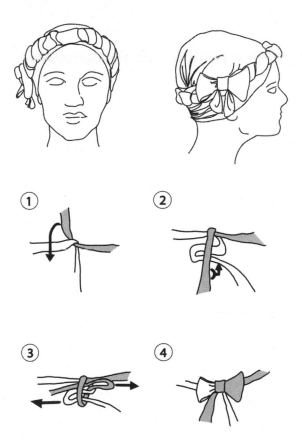

Bow

7. Tie ends in a half-knot.

8. Use lower tied end to form first loop.

9. Bring other end over and around first loop, continue partially through opening that is formed, thus making the knot and second loop.

10. Flare loops and spread center.

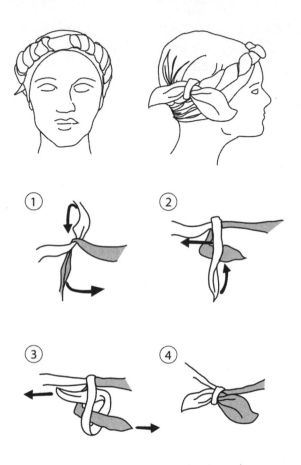

Square Knot

11. Tie half-knot.

12. Bring upper end down over lower piece.

13. Continue to loop around lower end and come through opening.

14. Flare endings and spread center knot.

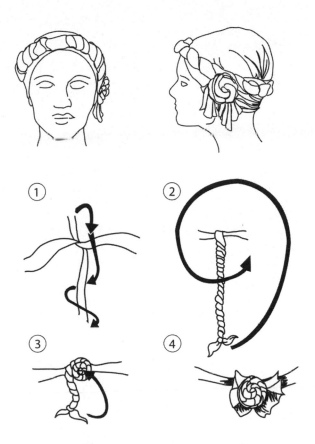

Rosette

15. Tie half-knot leaving ends long.

16. Intertwine ends tightly to form a coil, leaving a short length uncoiled.

17. Relax coil and guide it to encircle around itself flatly. Poke end of coil partially through center of circle.

18. Spread sash ends to ruffle around the rosette.

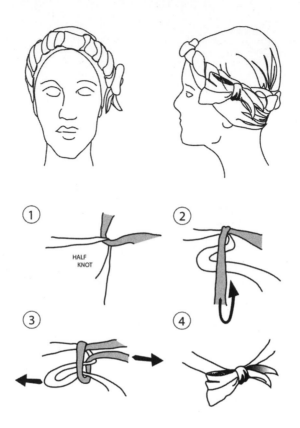

Half Bow

19. Tie ends in a half-knot with lower end twice as long as upper.

20. Use lower end to make a loop. Bring upper end down over loop.

21. Continue around lower loop and bring scarf end completely through opening.

22. Flare loop and spread knot.

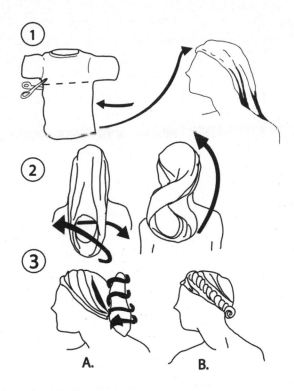

T-Shirt Wrap

A great idea for a casual spring or summer covering.

23. Cut straight across a T-shirt, just under the sleeves. There are now two pieces—the top ⅓ of the shirt (neck and sleeves) and a fabric "tube," which is the bottom ⅔.

24. Take the finished T-shirt hemline of the tube and place it centered on your forehead at the hairline.

25. At the back of the head, hold each side of the tube and cross the piece of fabric in the right hand over the left, creating a figure 8.

26. With the fabric crossed, pull the lower half of the figure 8 from the back of the head to the front, creating a halo or headband effect. Tuck in any loose fabric around the headband to create a neat look.

27. The final result will look like a cotton turban with a matching headband going around the head. T-shirt wraps may also be accented with fringe bangs.

28. The two sleeves of the top ⅓ may also be cut off and used as headbands.

You can use hats, baseball caps, or crazy, fun swimming caps to cover your baldness. Select ones with a fringe of hair at the bangs or along the back so that it appears as if you still are sporting a full head of hair. Or be bold, leave the head coverings in the closet, and face the world au natural.

"A woman can be bald, but that is more of a statement," Eivind says, while Oscar maintains that "a woman can look gorgeous without hair, as long as the shape of the skull is right. With the right shape and the right makeup, a very statuesque and spectacular look will result."

When the Shedding Starts

Depending on the type of chemotherapy you are receiving, your hair will start falling out about two weeks after the first cycle. If total hair loss is in your future, you will most likely face complete baldness by the second cycle.

"I always tell my friends to shave it off," Rick says. "Losing clumps of hair in the shower is traumatic. Don't give chemo that authority in your life. Shave it off and be done with it."

Because your hair will not fall out evenly, and coping can be very difficult, our experts agree that Rick's idea is the best approach.

Oribe remembers helping a friend once her hair started to fall out. "She had beautiful black hair and I shaved it for her. It was quite traumatic, but somehow empowering, watching her take her control back. It was summer, very hot, and one day I saw her sitting with her bald head. She was very comfortable with it. When her hair came back, it was as gorgeous and shiny and strong as ever."

Caring for Your Scalp

Once your hair is gone, you must treat your scalp gently.

"Stay away from abrasive products," Theresa says. "Treat your skin the way you would a baby's, using gentle cleansers."

Amy recommends using witch hazel to cleanse. Oribe suggests gentle massage to circulate the blood under the skin and help keep the hair follicles healthy. He also told us about a hair vitamin, Viviscal®, which he says all the top fashion models use.

"A lot of models have very thin hair, and it's burnt up and damaged and they swear by this vitamin," he explains. "They say Viviscal makes their hair stronger, shinier, and healthier. If it's okay with your doctor to take it, you may be helping your hair from the root out."

As with any advice you receive, research, or discover regarding your treatment, we urge you to discuss everything with your doctor. Do not take anything until your oncologist has specifically approved it.

Chemo Curls and Transitioning Back from Baldness

The moment your treatment ends, the drugs will begin to leave your body. Slowly your hair will return. It will grow in curly. For about a year you'll sport "chemo curls."

"They are gorgeous, simply incredible," Eivind says. "The women go out of here and they are all divas."

There's a period, maybe two months, when your hair's re-arrival is not ready for styling. The color may be depleted, dark gray, or sometimes white. It'll be super short, and what comes in may be a little on the fuzzy side. Don't worry; these are just the last of the hair cells burned by chemo drugs leaving your body to make way for the hair you've always known to come back. And it will—sometimes even better than before.

Until that happens, you still have got to get through this initial growing in. Our experts offer a variety of helpful options.

"Use gentle conditioners to combat the initial dryness," Oribe says. "Don't worry about cutting off the dead stuff as it comes in. I know most women want it to just grow in long, but if you can cut off the dry ends, and moisturize—olive oil is amazing—what you have will look healthier."

"Wait for a month or two," Eivind advises. "Then use low-peroxide, 2 percent or 3 percent, hair color. Read the ingredients list on the box to be sure you're buying the gentlest product. Dilute it by half with water. Leave it on for a few minutes and then shampoo it for a few minutes, just to put some color there."

"Doing a vegetable rinse or a semipermanent color is a

good idea," Oribe agrees. "It gives the new hair depth and makes it look young and healthy."

When the curls begin to form, Oribe says the best styles are easy, boyish cuts. "You're always fighting roundness with curly hair. You have to sculpt it a bit. You have to cheat a little bit. It doesn't grow in evenly. You can play with it, change it around.

"You want a haircut that sort of feathers and layers, so that you can place it where the hair is not growing back as full," Theresa says. "The look is sort of fringy and easy.

"You have to work with your hairdresser," Oribe advises. "Figure out a game plan, how you're going to grow it in, and work on a style that lets you take advantage of what is happening with your natural growth."

Finding Your Hair Helper

Working with a hairdresser ready to be your partner as you transition back from baldness is a great benefit, but if you don't already have a wonderful stylist, how can you find such a person to help you?

Our experts insist that hair and beauty professionals will do whatever they can to assist a chemo girl, as long as they understand what she is facing and what she needs.

"It's very important to find a hairdresser who is kind and willing to be gentle with you and your hair," Oribe says. "Ask friends for recommendations. Go to a local salon. Talk to the manager. Ask which of the stylists is the most artistic. Explain what is happening to you. Ask which is the most visual—who would be the most artistic when it comes to cutting a wig and patient enough to help you style your very short hair."

Walk into a salon, and tell the receptionist you want to get a sense of the atmosphere. Watch the different cutters to feel out which have the temperament you would feel most comfortable with.

Deann says trust your instincts. "You should feel relaxed and comfortable and cared for. It's like choosing your doctor. You need a good rapport with the person who will be caring for you. If something doesn't feel right, move on."

"On a karmic level, I believe everyone who comes to me is there to teach me something," says Amy. "One of my jobs is to help take away the fear and sense of loss and replace it with the feeling that they are beautiful from the inside out. I show them the opportunities they still have to look good. I want them to leave my studio ready to get through the experience with strength and hope and a positive result. What you believe more times than not is what you create."

Most wig salon employees will understand your situation and will be ready to help. Since Hasidic women often wear wigs, you will find both wig and hair salons that are very adept at fulfilling your needs in those communities.

If you cannot connect with a wigmaker locally or online, Amy, Deann, and Eivind regularly work with women long distance and can ship custom wigs anywhere in the world.

The process is fairly simple. Clients contact the salon, send pictures of themselves in their natural hair, and include magazine clippings of styles they like. A long phone call follows, fleshing out the details of style, color, and cut.

"They send or e-mail pictures," Deann explains. "They talk to me about what they like and don't like. I listen very carefully. It's amazing. Our mail-order clients are as happy with the style and the fit of their wigs as those who come into the salon."

Amy, Deann, Eivind, Oribe, Oscar, Rick, and Theresa want you to remember that all the people who work in their industries have dedicated their professional lives to helping women look beautiful. Help is just a question away. If you muster up the courage to talk with stylists about what is happening to you, they will most likely do all they can to assist you in your quest for normalcy during an extremely tough time.

"They say there are three people a woman talks to when she's diagnosed with cancer," Eivind says. "Her God, her husband, and her cosmetologist."

Open up to beauty professionals about your situation. You will be greeted with open arms. If you are brave enough to ask for assistance, you will be rewarded with compassion, understanding, and hands-on help. Reach out for help, and you will see that even though you are sick, you are not alone. You can be brave, and you will be beautiful.

For more information about the material presented in this chapter, please visit the following websites:

www.lookgoodfeelbetter.org

www.amyspresence.com

www.oribesalon.com

www.oscarblandi.com/salon.html

www.wigsbytiffany.com

www.internationalhairgoods.com

www.discoverspas.com/Washington_DC/dclucien.shtml

www.viviscal.com

CHAPTER 3

Skin Deep

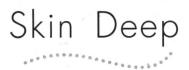

THE SURVIVORS REMEMBER

Marybeth: My skin became very dry and pallid, but I didn't experience many of the more challenging side effects. My face was another story. Without eyebrows or lashes to offset my eyes, I looked almost transparent. My wig's bangs concealed some of the problem, and I lived in lipstick because with my lips done and my wig on, all I needed was a pair of sunglasses to go outside with minimum effort looking totally normal.

Chris: I lost my eyelashes, I lost my eyebrows, I was completely, totally bald, and I had a face full of pimples! I dealt with these issues as best I could by always wearing makeup and keeping my skin clean and moisturized. I also wore a lot of black. I thought it was flattering, slimming, and made me look more elegant and put together than I felt.

Laura: It was very important to me to try to look pretty while going through my treatment. It was a statement I chose to make as if I was saying, "This is not going to get me down." I needed to wear eyeliner but my eyes became very sensitive and watered easily, so finding the right eye makeup was a challenge. My skin was yellow and I had dark rings under my eyes that I tried to correct with natural-looking foundation.

Patricia: I didn't lose my eyebrows and eyelashes until I began the Taxol phase of my treatment, but it was very important to me not to look sick. Once they were gone, I went right to Elizabeth Arden and had a cosmetologist teach me how to draw on eyebrows and recreate the illusion of lashes.

Rosemarie: I couldn't draw on brows and didn't bother trying to replace my lashes. It just wasn't me. I did buy every color lip gloss. My sister and I would go shopping and I'd look for new brands, new shades. Playing up my lips was easy, and it made me feel good.

The Pearls

Next to hair, our face and skin stand on the front lines of chemo. They are the most noticeable victims of the chemical assault, done in by their cells' propensity to multiply rapidly.

Depending on how your body reacts to treatment, you may find yourself batting lashless eyes, raising missing brows, or cracking a smile through thirsty lips. Your skin may become red or flaky. Steroids may produce a crop of pimples. The whites of your eyes may develop an odd yellow or bluish tint. Your complexion may turn sallow or ashy.

The Side Effects/Face

lost eyebrows	dryness
lost eyelashes	flushed face
dry lips	yellow or blue tint to
sallow skin	whites of eyes
irregular pigmentation	acne
redness	

The Side Effects/Skin

rashes (itchy and	redness
nonitchy)	thickening
irregular pigmentation	dryness
extreme sun sensitivity	sunburn-type pain

Because skin cells are dying so rapidly, some chemo girls' medication induces a never-ending exfoliation, so that instead of problems with your skin, you may enjoy an absolutely glowing epidermis from first cycle to last.

Unlike hair, which either stays or falls out, your skin is subject to a variety of potential side effects. There's literally no way to know which will happen to you before chemotherapy starts. Your doctor will give you a general guideline, but until you go through a cycle or two, you won't really know what's in store for your face and skin.

Even if you escape many of the tougher side effects, there are still things you can do to make yourself look and feel better.

"In my experience, most women want to know what they can do to perk themselves up," says Academy Award–winning makeup artist Michele Burke. "It's not about looking the same as they did before. It's a question of how to take what they've got and make it their personal best regardless of the changes they're experiencing."

Theresa Loupuchin agrees. "Our face and skin are two of the most visible aspects of our bodies. This is all about empowerment. If lipstick or body butter is going to boost our morale and make us feel healthier, why not go for it?"

We hope you'll be one of the chemo girls who glides through her treatment without changes to your skin. But if you wake up one morning and notice that your eyes look different, or you have some discoloration on your cheeks, or your skin feels like it's a half size too tight, fear not. Our experts have drawn on their years of hands-on experience to create a game plan to help you pull through.

WHAT'S GOING ON

A hair cell is a hair cell, whether it grows under your arms, inside your nose, or across your brow. If the hair on your head begins to fall out, be prepared to face a similar loss everywhere else, including your face.

With zillions of skin cells providing a rapidly dividing bull's-eye for chemo's arrows, it's no wonder our outer shell suffers.

"The skin is the largest organ of the body, connected to every other organ through the blood vessels, and its role is to protect us and our organs," says internationally renowned dermatologist Dr. Howard Murad. "When the body experiences chemotherapy, the skin's barrier can be compromised. The result is redness, dryness, itching, or overall sensitivity."

Our embattled sweat glands secrete less oil, triggering dryness from our forehead to our feet. More times than not, steroids are to blame for breakouts, while irregular pigmentation and darkened skin are due to the effects of the sun.

"The underlying derma barrier is impaired during chemo," says aesthetician and skin care expert Krista Dibsie. "You have to strengthen that layer, keep the blood circulating, and replenish what's been stripped by chemicals."

"You need treatment in order to become well," says celebrity dermatologist Dr. Patricia Wexler, "but just because you're on chemotherapy does not mean you cannot or should not treat the symptoms that are causing emotional pain."

Don't be afraid to take back your face and skin if they begin to fold under the chemo attack.

The Basics—Cleansing, Moisturizing, Protecting

Now more than ever, you must treat your skin very kindly. Your standard skin care steps won't change in any significant way during treatment. You'll still cleanse and moisturize but will have to concentrate on keeping the skin calm and protected from the elements.

"During chemo, your skin is in a raw state," explains Estée Lauder executive vice president Harvey Gedeon. "You must stay away from anything that may elicit a reaction. Use products whose ingredients are extremely gentle—no detergents, no color, or fragrance."

"Chemo reduces your resistance," says Theresa, "and you don't fight things off as well as you once did, so you want to keep germs and bacteria away from your skin."

"If you were clean before," she adds, "you have to be even cleaner now."

Cleansing Your Face . . .

The key to successful cleansing is to select mild, moisturizing, nonabrasive products manufactured specifically for sensitive skin.

"Cleansing can be very harsh," says Harvey. "It opens everything up, making your skin vulnerable to other problems. We always recommend a gentle cleanser without any detergents."

"I like the milky cleansers best," says Michele. "Use them like ordinary soap, lathering and then washing off with warm water. You should do it in steps—wash, rinse, pat gently with a soft cloth to make sure that all traces are gone, and have a good final rinse."

Louis Philippe DeMontpensier, who Jacqueline Kennedy Onassis turned to during her cancer battle, prefers creamy, water-soluble products, and recommends against using any sort of paper on your face. "I recommend against cleansers that must be wiped away because the tissues tend to leave little traces of pulp on the skin. You want to be able to wash your cleanser off with water."

Theresa agrees. "Tissues can be abrasive. If you're going to wipe your skin, use a soft, one hundred percent cotton cloth."

Theresa also cautions against the use of soap. "While in treatment, forget about using soap. Instead, stick with the nonsoap cleansers and stay away from gels, which contain alcohol and are drying."

Your shopping habits don't need to change because of your condition. If you've always picked up your beauty products at the grocery or drug store, you will still find exactly what you need there, while women who enjoy buying their cosmetics and cleansers from a department store may continue to visit their favorite counters.

"No matter what their financial situation, everybody buys things at their local drug store," Theresa says. "You don't need to go spending a lot of money. There are plenty of wonderful, quality products available at whatever price range you find most comfortable."

Michele says, "Any brand that is tried and true and that you know has been tested forever in the labs will work very well. Just check the ingredients list to be sure it has what you want, and stay away from scents and other ingredients that may be too harsh."

Harvey cautions chemo girls to buy only from trustworthy sources. "Unknown lines, or products that are so-called all natural, may cause more harm than good," he explains. "You must be careful. After all, poison ivy is very natural, and lemon is very natural. On hypersensitive skin, even these all-natural products could cause harm."

. . . and Your Body

Just as with your face, you should stay away from body soaps or cleansers that contain alcohol, oil, fragrance, or harsh chemicals. Avoid deodorant soaps until treatment ends. Instead, pick up a mild soap or body wash without fragrance, oil, or alcohol. To minimize dryness, keep your bathing time short.

"Don't take long showers, and don't soak in the tub," advises Dr. Wexler. "Use lukewarm water, not hot, and then towel dry and moisturize while your skin is still damp."

"It's all about hydration," says Theresa. "Putting oils in the bathwater won't help because they can cause yeast infections. Stay out of the tub, stick to the shower, and forget about the loofahs and scrubbys until your treatment is over."

If you're itchy, stay away from oils and instead choose a heavier cream made for sensitive skin, Krista advises. "Smooth it everywhere, even your back, before you go to sleep. You'll be so much more comfortable during the night."

Moisturizing Your Face . . .

Once your skin is clean and slightly damp, apply fragrance-free, oil-free, alcohol-free moisturizer.

"Choose a water-based moisturizer with a high SPF," says Louis Philippe. "You don't want to overmoisturize, so apply it lightly, in thin layers. The process needs to even the skin's texture, so when you put on foundation, the dry spots on your skin don't soak up whatever oil is in the product, and stand out on your face."

"Here's the trick," he says. "Apply a layer, and if after thirty seconds it feels taut, then put on another, until your skin is supple and comfortable."

Dr. Murad recommends facial moisturizers with antioxidants as an effective way to hydrate and even skin tone. "Look for vitamin C, vitamin E, grapeseed extracts, or green tea," he says.

Michele is also a fan of antioxidants and botanicals. "Shea butter, avocado, anything with olive oil or seaweed. You really can't get better than that."

Harvey suggests looking at the ingredients list for the type of sunscreen being used. "You want a good SPF. We recommend nonchemical products that will sit on the skin and not penetrate."

Nonchemical sunscreens usually contain titanium dioxide or zinc oxide or both, two nonirritating ingredients that are ideal for use on all skin types, and Harvey recommends looking for those "mechanical blockers."

If you do have a reaction to something you've put on, "Take it off," says Louis Philippe. "If it tingles or feels uncomfortable, your skin doesn't like it. Just wash it off and start again."

. . . and Your Body

Any moisturizer that makes your skin feel soft and supple will work well for chemo girls, though our experts were partial to creams and recommended against oils.

"I don't find oils to be good emollients because they don't add moisture, they just seal it in," says Dr. Wexler. "If you don't have any moisture to begin with, they're not helping."

"I'm a big fan of body butters," notes Theresa. "It feels

so good to put creamy things on and luxuriate in them as you rub your skin."

Dr. Wexler says any emollient will work. "You can use anything that is healing and nourishing. Vitamin E, aloe, chamomile, and arnica will all help relieve dry, flaky skin."

"Look for hydrating products that attract water and hold it in the skin," advises Dr. Murad. "Sodium PCA, hyaluronic acid, sorbitol, algae extract, and various plant-based lipids like avocado oil are all good hydrators."

Apply moisturizing products whenever your skin is in need of relief.

"Your skin isn't reacting normally while you're on chemo," says Dr. Wexler. "It can get very dry and very raw, and it can be very uncomfortable. You want to treat it kindly and be very gentle. Keep moisturizing, and don't exfoliate if it's red or stressed. It will need time to heal."

To Peel or Not to Peel—Exfoliation, Toners, and Astringents

If you find that your skin becomes excessively flaky or rough, mild, gentle products formulated for dry, adult, or sensitive skin may help alleviate these conditions.

"If you don't overdo it, mild exfoliation is fine," says Dr. Murad. "It will help keep the skin hydrated as well, since the dehydrated cells are removed."

"If you select a system that contains microabrasion with aluminum oxide crystals, or glycolic acids or fruity acids, made for very sensitive skin, you should be fine," Dr. Wexler says.

If your skin is turning rough or creased, "A gentle exfoliate with a mild scrub or a cleanser with jojoba beads and some mild alpha hydroxy acids is fine," Dr. Murad says. "You can also use a textured washcloth to buff away surface skin cells that build up."

It is essential to apply moisturizer immediately after exfoliation, but there are times and conditions where even the gentlest exfoliation must be avoided.

"Never exfoliate radiated skin," Dr. Wexler says, "because it's essentially burned, and it's going to be much thinner than skin that hasn't been photodamaged."

Regardless of your skin's texture or the gentleness of your product, use common sense.

"Don't exfoliate to the point of causing soreness or abrasion," Dr. Wexler says. "Keep it gentle and moisturize, moisturize, moisturize."

Likewise, fans of astringents and toners should keep their selections to the mild side of the product spectrum.

"I usually forgo toners because they can be too drying," says Michele, "but if you use one, it should be gentle, like a rosewater, or one with seaweed. If your skin is on the greasy side, a little witch hazel is very gentle and good."

"If you're using astringents with alcohol, please stop," says Theresa. "Put those products away and maintain a skin care regime that is not harsh, nonabrasive, and extremely mild."

Protecting Your Skin from the Sun

If there is one rule for chemo girls it is this: stay out of the sun.

Sunlight will damage even the healthiest skin, and photosensitized chemotherapy skin is at a heightened risk for burns, spots, discolorations, and uneven pigmentation.

"You really have to be careful about sun exposure and very proactive about your sunscreen," Dr. Wexler says. "Wear a UVA/UVB protection every day with a minimum SPF 30 every time you go outside."

Dr. Murad stresses several important sunscreen points. "Even when it's cloudy, UVA and UVB rays reach their way into your skin," he says. "You must use sunscreen year round."

"Apply one ounce (or two tablespoons) to your entire body at least 30 minutes before going outdoors," he continues. "Wear tightly woven fabrics or clothing that is labeled with an Ultraviolet Protection Factor (UPF). You can even wash sunscreen into your clothing with laundry powders such as SunGuard, which provides protection up to 20 washings per garment."

Lightly colored or loosely woven clothing offers little protection against the sun's powerful rays. According to the Skin Cancer Foundation, a T-shirt has an SPF of 7, while a dark, tightly woven denim shirt has an SPF of 1,700.

While it may not be realistic to wear dark, heavier clothing in the warmer climates, there are other options for protecting your chemo-sensitive skin from the sun.

"If you're a golfer, play the first round," Theresa says. "If tennis or walking is your thing, go early, before the sun is too strong, or later in the evening, if you're not too tired."

Be sensible about the timing of your outdoor activities, avoiding the strongest rays, which generally shine between 11 A.M. and 4 P.M.

Mechanical blockers such as zinc oxide and titanium dioxide are preferable to chemical sunscreens because they lie on top of the skin and do not penetrate.

"You can also use mineral powders," Theresa says, though Dr. Wexler warns that they, too, can be irritating. "Some say mechanical blockers are less irritating than chemical, but if the SPF is not high enough and you end up using more, or experiencing a burn, that can be irritating or damaging."

"It's trial and error," Dr. Wexler says. "Use whatever works best for you, but use it every day of the year."

Hello, Face!

Now that you have your skin clean and moisturized and protected, you can begin to play with makeup, restoring with your powders, brushes, and creams any features chemo may have temporarily compromised.

When it comes to makeup, Rick DiCecca sums up a chemo girl's dilemma. "Whether or not she considers herself beautiful, society judges a woman by the way she looks. When that is taken away because of chemotherapy, it's a very frightening place to be.

"I see my job as helping her rediscover her beauty," Rick continues. "It may not exactly match her perception of what she had before, but whatever the problem, there is a solution, and by helping clients realize this, I hope to give them their power back."

Our makeup artists and cosmetologists believe that there is no face-related, chemo-induced side effect that cosmetics cannot effectively resolve.

"It is very satisfying to help people who are still in shock about their diagnosis to understand that their beauty problems are only temporary," says Louis Philippe. "Once we begin working with them, the help is spiritual as well as physical. I transform their faces, and they see that they can look better, and they immediately begin to feel better about themselves."

Anastasia of Beverly Hills believes all women facing chemo are heroes. "It can be very traumatic, but I encourage them always to remember that there is no need to be afraid of what will happen. Mental strength is the most important thing, but knowing that there are makeup tricks definitely helps."

Whether you're just learning what your protocol will be or are already deep in the chemo trenches, take heart. There are ways to correct whatever may be causing you unhappiness with the way you look. Step by step, our experts have outlined what you can do to look your personal best until your treatment is over and your face—and life—are once again your own.

Step 1: Look in the Mirror

With a long career in the movie business, Michele knows when looking at a person's face, the camera—and the eye—focus on one key feature.

"I call it the magic trick," she says. "When people look at you, they're going to look at one thing. Usually it's your eyes or your lips. You want them to focus on what you have that's amazing still and not on what you want to hide."

"Even if you don't have lashes, you can line your eyes with a soft pencil, add some eyebrows, and put a soft shadow on the lids," she explains. "If you've got dark circles or your skin is really sallow, get a great lipstick—you'll be amazed at how much a bright, shiny color on your mouth will accentuate your eyes and enhance your overall complexion."

Rick agrees. "Draw attention to your best feature and make it pop," he says. Louis Philippe reminds chemo girls to avoid trying too hard to conceal an obvious problem. "You can call more attention to the problem than make it look better," he says. "You don't want to look too painted or forced. You want to look natural."

Take some time to assess yourself. Decide what on your face is still as wonderful as ever, and then work your makeup routine around that attribute. Once you've identified your best facial feature, you're well on your way toward projecting yourself as a woman who isn't preoccupied with illness, but rather a person who is dealing with her changing sense of beauty, well groomed and ready to put her best foot forward.

Foundation. Foundations should only be applied to cleaned, moisturized skin. They should be alcohol and fragrance free and, if possible, formulated especially for sensitive skin. You may find one with a sunscreen that will help block out pollution and sunlight, though Theresa warns that depending on a foundation to provide you with adequate sun protection is not wise.

"Foundation wears off during the day, and the sunscreen will dissipate and not protect you," she says. "You want to apply your sunscreen as either a separate product or with your moisturizer. If you get a tinted moisturizer with an SPF 30, you've now applied your protection and given yourself some color. Three quarters of the job is done."

When selecting a foundation shade, Theresa explains the standard test for getting the right color: "Stripe your skin at the jawline. If there's a line of demarcation between your jaw and your neck, you have got the wrong color. Depending on the result of the test, try a step up or down until you find the shade that most closely matches your own."

"If you're at a cosmetics counter, you can try all the shades until you find the one that is right for you," says Michele. "Even if you don't want to buy their products, most of the consultants will be happy to help you if you can muster up the courage to tell them what you're dealing with. You can take samples of the colors that work best to a mass market retailer and try to match them to a packaged foundation."

Because drugstore and grocery-store makeup is sealed, Michele recommends picking up a shade that is warmer than your sample and another that is cooler than your sample; then mix them up to get the perfect color.

"Quite often I'll do a drop of warm and a drop of cool, because some of the warmer colors are too orangey and the cooler colors are too white, when what you need is a little of each to make the shade that will work best for you."

Some foundations feature ingredients that can help camouflage the appearance of dryness. "Smooth, well-hydrated
skin reflects light and makes your skin look healthy," Rick
says. "But, of course, chemo skin is not smooth or well hydrated, so the trick is to pick skin-illuminating bases and
concealers that brighten and balance skin tone while helping to hide flaws."

"Look for face products that create illumination; there
is an ingredient called gransil, a microscopic silicone that
creates iridescence."

You can also try mineral powders. Brush them on and
you have both your sunblock and foundation covered.

To apply a liquid foundation, use a dry cosmetic sponge
and stipple on the color by putting a bit on the sponge and
then pressing it onto your skin, then flicking your wrist,
bringing the sponge away.

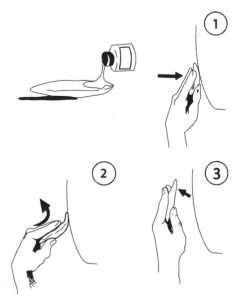

"Imagine you're sponge painting your face," Theresa says. "Blend the product in, rather than poking or jabbing or rubbing."

"While the skin is still slightly damp, dot the foundation anywhere you think you'll need it, like the T-zone, under the eyes, and around the mouth," says Michele. "Don't forget your throat and chin. Once you feel it's all blended, look and see where the discolorations or other problems are, and then go back in with a concealer."

Concealer. If you've got dark circles under your eyes, uneven pigmentation on your cheeks, pimples, or dark spots on your skin, a concealer will help cover up the problem.

"Concealer is usually a product with more density than foundation," explains Louis Philippe. Keeping in mind his advice not to overdo your coverage, he recommends selecting a concealer that is one step up from your foundation color.

"If you're trying to cover something on your skin that is darker than your regular complexion, you need a lighter concealer, a liquid or compact," he says. "I use an acrylic brush, not a regular makeup brush, and I apply it in thin layers until you see less and less and less."

Michele finds fingers are very useful for covering spots. "You can blend the concealer in by dotting it on and then lightly tapping it with your finger to blend it," she says. "Then get another dot of foundation and dot that, and then a powder that you blot on top. Usually that's enough."

Michele urges restraint when trying to camouflage irregularities in the skin. "If you try to overcompensate and hide every little blemish and problem, you may end up looking worse," she says. "You don't want to look like you tried too hard. A good foundation, carefully applied, is usually plenty."

Blush. Pale or sallow skin needs a bit of perking up. Blushers will not only provide color to your face but will also brighten the appearance of your eyes and help draw attention away from any trouble that you may be experiencing with your skin.

"Just a splash at the top of the cheekbones is all you need," says Michele. "Adding a tiny bit to the brow bone really makes the eyes look good—put it just below the brow, going up to the forehead. Then smile, add a bit more to the apples of your cheeks, and watch how it will brighten your appearance, making you look less drawn."

When selecting a color, Michele likes peach or soft pinks for light skins, plums or rose for medium skins, and plumy browns or bronze, copper, or brick-hued colors for darker skin. Our experts preferred powders to creams or gels, since they can be loosely brushed over prepared skin, then lightly blended with a cotton ball or soft cloth.

Theresa reminds chemo girls about cleanliness with your brushes during treatment, saying, "If you're not using disposable applicators, prevent bacteria build up by regularly washing your brushes with shampoo and letting them air dry overnight."

"Don't use antibacterial soap or alcohol to clean them," she advises. "They're too harsh and will damage the fibers."

Lips.   While opinions may differ as to which facial feature is usually the most compelling, in the contest between eyes and lips, chemo seems to give a distinct advantage to our mouths.

"Lipstick is the biggest selling product in the industry," says Louis Philippe. "The secret is to pick the shade that's going to make your eyes look better."

"Look for a good moisturizer with emollients, like lanolin," he advises. "As to color, it's really your own personal preference. Make sure it has a high SPF, of course, and go for a glossy, translucent shade that looks dewy and hydrated."

Theresa agrees. "Matte isn't a great look during chemo," she says. "It tends to be too drying. I recommend finding a balm with vitamin E or shea butter, and staying with the same colors you love, just going more for a gloss."

Michele says a balm and a gloss used together work wonders. "My favorite thing to use on lips is an all natural balm, then cover with a bright pigment. You'll get a nice color with a shiny, hydrated, creamy finish that is quite becoming."

Krista says don't forget the sunscreen. "Lips are just as exposed to UVA and UVB as the rest of our face. It's important to keep them moisturized and protected with the same SPF we use on our face. Don't use too much lipstick or chapstick—they seal in moisture, but once the product dissipates, your lips become moisture depleted. Instead, get a good hydrating serum."

If your lips suffer, Dr. Murad says, "An ointment with petroleum, vitamin E, and salicylic acid is ideal. Look for formulas with at least an SPF 15."

Step 2: All About Eyes

They are called the window to our souls, and during chemo, our eyes can reflect a tale of hardship, but they can also remain one of our best features.

"Chemotherapy will not change your eye color," says Louis Philippe, "so you can enhance that natural color by selecting the right shades to work with."

"If you have green eyes, go for lavender, or any color that makes your eyes look greener," he explains. "If your eyes are blue, go for browns, and if your eyes are brown, pick a navy blue. These shades will accentuate all the natural beauty of your eyes and make working with them a lot of fun."

Michele says taupe is a wonderful color for almost any skin type, along with soft grays and browns. She recommends against shimmers or pearls because of the dryness in your skin.

"Your water retention is off when you're ill," she says, "So shimmers and pearls are no good because they can bring out the crêpe texture on the lids.

"Remember," Michele says, "one of the best tricks for the eyes is to use the right blush. When color is applied on the brow bone and the cheeks, your eyes will look really good."

Lashes.   If you've lost your lashes, several simple makeup tricks are available that you can use to make your eyes look more like they always have. Under our lashes, there is a rim of dark skin, which most of us never see, since the lashes cover it. The first step to filling in the look of lashes is to cover that darker rim.

"Use an eye shadow base or a concealer on the lid to even out the color," says Theresa. "Take a little brush and apply it to the upper and lower rim of the eyes, and gently blend it in. That will automatically get rid of that red, tired look."

Next, you simply have to darken the edge of your lids, to recreate the hue of lashes.

"Most of us don't have very long lashes," Theresa explains. "That's why mascara is so popular—it makes what we have look darker and longer. If your lashes have fallen out, depending on the color of your skin, all you need to do is get a brown or black eyeliner and dot it along the lash line with a little brush or Q-tip and blend that. It will create the darkness at the base of the lashes, maintaining the illusion that your lashes are not missing."

"Concentrate on the top lash," advises Louis Philippe. "Get a liquid or pencil eyeliner and use just a little bit, carefully blended in, to give your eye form and definition."

Going false.   Regularly using false eyelashes during treatment can irritate the skin around your eyes. Therefore, apply false eyelashes only if a special occasion requires special intervention.

"Lashes are there to protect our eyes," Theresa explains. "If they're gone, you've lost that protection, and you want to be careful. You don't want foreign material like glue on your skin, which is already thinner because of treatment. You don't want to be pulling the lashes off and straining the skin."

That said, everyone understands that sometimes eyelashes are a feature chemo girls don't want to be without.

"If you're going out to an event and you don't want people remarking on the way you look, then buy the lashes that come in a strip," Michele says. "Select the type that look natural and subdued, with paler fibers and just a few hairs on them," she says. "You get an applicator and directions in the package. Once you've got them on, add some shadow to the root of the lash line with a brush so they don't look fake."

Stay with soft grays, browns, and taupe shadows, Michele advises. Avoid light blue, green, or dark black.

"You don't want to look like a Vegas dancer," she cautions. "You want the look to be the least flamboyant, most natural you can achieve."

If you're shopping for lashes, Rick says that you can get an idea of what looks most natural by looking in the mass market at the Ardell brand style #124 or the Andrea brand #53. He said that department store shoppers can visit the M-A-C counter for ideas on what's available and looks best for their face.

The shades you pick to outline your eyes will have a lot to do with how well they look when you're finished putting your lashes on.

"It's all about contrasting the colors to compliment your eye," says Louis Philippe. "If your eyes are dark blue, your liners and shadows can be orangey or reddish brown," he says. "If they're dark brown, navy is just gorgeous.

"Cover the line where the lashes were, or shadow over the line where the lash strip lies," he says. "Create your eye shape with the color, then at the outer edge of your lid, pull the line slightly upward. This will defy gravity, making you look refreshed, not tired."

Louis Philippe says when doing makeup, the trick is to keep the application moving up, not down.

"Don't add to the pull of gravity," he advises. "Always keep your motions moving upward."

Brows.   Missing brows can be covered by a wig's bangs or sunglasses. You can draw them on with a pencil or stencil them on with powder.

When it comes to brow beauty, perhaps no one is more renowned for her expertise than Anastasia of Beverly Hills, who offers a variety of stencil kits and products to help a chemo girl replace her missing brows.

When considering stencils, Anastasia says the best choice for all women without any brows on her face is a smaller, medium width brow (like the Petite stencil in her line). If there are still some brows on your face, she recommends following the package instructions, but if the brow is completely missing, Anastasia advises applying a colorless gel within the stencil first to help grab and hold onto the colored powder.

When choosing a brow shade, Michele says, "You don't want it to be too intense," she explains. "Go for something two to three shades lighter than your natural hair color. If you're using a stencil, put it in place and color it in; then, if it seems like it's too much, use your compact and a powder puff to dust over it to bring the color back."

Drawing on eyebrows is another simple solution. A bit

of practice and the right shade will more than compensate for any strangeness you may feel should your brows become sparse or disappear altogether.

"The trick is to draw the line in short strokes, using a pencil that is ash or dark brown if your skin is dark or matching to a shade lighter than your natural brow color if your complexion is lighter," says Louis Philippe.

"I would stay away from black, even if your hair is black," Michele says, "because it's just too dark, too intense."

"I like dark brown, taupe, auburn—something that is soft and looks natural and not too contrasting," she says. "Etch it along in little strokes and then pat down with some compact powder. Put them on after the foundation, so you have a better sense of how much color you want there."

Drawing on brows.   This is a simple, four-step process:

1. Place a thin pencil along the side of your nose and make a small dot where the brow should begin. Make that point 1.
2. Move the pencil so that it lines up with the outer edge of the pupil. Mark that spot with a small dot. Make that point 2.

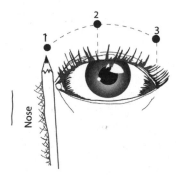

3. Lower the pencil so that it's lying along the outer edge of the eye. Mark a small dot there (point 3).

4. Start with point 1 and use short strokes with a brow pencil to connect to point 2. This is the start of your brow shape. Continue to apply brow pencil, creating a thicker area closest to your nose and make it thinner toward the end.

Applying a stencil.   Purchase a stencil kit from any drugstore, grocery store, makeup counter, or online source. Follow the package directions.

Tints.   If your treatment is triggering a blue or yellow tint to the whites of your eyes, clever use of color will help take away some of the effect.

"Think of the color wheel," says Theresa. "Go for the contrast that will lessen the look of what's happening. If you're yellow, stay away from browns. Use soft black or gray black. You can find a colorwheel on our website www.beauty pearlsforchemogirls.com. That will help offset the tint and make the whites look whiter."

Darker-skinned women generally experience more of the yellow tint, while fairer-toned women may see the whites of their eyes tinged with blue.

"If it's blue, go for taupe or soft browns," Theresa recommends. Anastasia agrees that warm tones will help offset the blueness.

"You can go for one of the pencils with a little sparkle in it," says Michele, "Lightly etch and trace the outline of the eye, and then with your finger, smudge the color. You don't want to emphasize the eye in this situation, but you do want to play down the unusual color."

Sunken eyes.   Ever the optimist, Theresa says that the best way to look at sunken eyes is to recast them as deep set.

"Now it's not a problem," she explains. "It's just another feature we want to make look its best."

Since the problem is fighting darkness, Theresa says you need to use the law of nature. "Put light on it. Use cream-colored eye shadows, peach-colored eye shadows, and soft white. Cream is the universal forgiveness color. It works for anybody."

"Brighten and conceal," Rick says. "Don't do too much. Let another part of your face dominate if your eyes aren't looking great."

Dark circles.   It's rare not to experience dark circles some time during treatment. Fortunately, the solutions are fairly simple to implement.

"Use light colors, a lighter shade of concealer, and eye shadow," says Anastasia.

"Take your compact or liquid concealer and apply it lightly with a little acrylic brush," says Louis Philippe. "Do a thin layer, step back and look, and then reapply in thin layers until you have the coverage you want."

Michele reminds us that the key to making up our chemo face is no different from making up our perfectly healthy face: by defining what works and by not worrying so much about perceived flaws.

"The eye of the observer does not really see what you're worried about," she says. "Pop what you think is the best feature, and the eye will naturally go to that feature."

Step 3: Dealing with Skin-Related Side Effects

If your chemo triggers skin-related side effects, there are a few things to remember:

- Understand that these effects are only temporary. The problem will ebb and finally disappear once your treatment ends.

- Be aware that there are solutions for any problem. Don't let a spot or pimple ruin your day. An imperfection that seems enormous to you may be almost invisible to those looking at you. Do whatever you need to do to feel comfortable and confident, but be kind to yourself. Your goal here shouldn't be trying to look like a fashion model (unless you are one). Just do whatever you can to feel good during a challenging time.

- Talk to your doctor about your side effects. Make sure there isn't an underlying issue, such as an allergic reaction, that is causing your face or skin to change. Communicate any problems, concerns, or issues you are facing to your health-care team. They are the professionals you should turn to for guidance and instruction on how to cope with your side effects. And if they say don't worry, then don't.

Sallowness.   Sallow skin color often occurs during chemo treatment. Improve the color of your skin by moving away from yellow-based products and using those with more pink or bronze in them.

"You want a little pink, but not too much because then it looks chalky," says Theresa. "You want to lift the skin color. Primers with opalescence, a little bit of pinkness in the shade, work wonders.

"You can use a tinted moisturizer," she says, "just stay away from the yellows. If you like bronzer, select one with more of a pink undertone than gold."

Dr. Wexler reminds chemo girls to watch what they eat. "Avoid the more vitamin A–rich veggies, like carrots and squash, which are just going to add to the problem. Supplement your diet with vegetables that won't contribute to the overall yellowness in your skin."

Ashiness.   Women of color may find their skin turning ashy as treatment continues. The condition is their skin's way of dealing with the dryness, so mild exfoliation and peels may help, along with careful cleansing and moisturizing.

"Use a damp cotton pad while cleansing to help remove the dead skin cells," Theresa advises. "Then moisturize and apply a foundation that will boost the color of the skin."

Because there are about fifty potential shades available to darker-skinned women, making the right choice in coverage shade can be daunting.

"Look for copper or burgundy undertones," Theresa says. "If you have the time and the access, go to a department store's cosmetics counter and work with the women there to find the best shade for you."

Redness/flushing.   You may be sitting comfortably at your desk, or doing something in the house, or perhaps driving along in your car, and suddenly your face will flush. This is usually a harmless rosacea, and there are a variety of ways to treat the condition.

"Most topical rosacea products like azelaic acid, sodium sulfacetamide, and topical metronidazole are fine," says Dr. Wexler. "Salicylic acid is also good."

"Facial regimens with goji berry extract and additional skin-soothing ingredients will help with the redness," Dr. Murad says, while Harvey adds that an anti-inflammatory cream will do wonders.

"The redness is hypersensitivity and inflammation," he says. "Look for ingredients that will calm the skin—vitamin C, vitamin E, anything that will provide redness relief."

"Massage will help with circulation and keep the skin tone even," says Krista. "Look for calming ingredients like lavender and chamomile, or find a serum that contains vitamin K, an antioxidant that calms the capillaries."

"Never be rough with your skin," advises Theresa. "If you're very sensitive, avoid products with oil. If you normally use astringents, toners, or other drying products, put them away until your treatment is over."

"If my patients are having a problem, I put them on a treatment of Minocin or tetracycline," says Dr. Wexler. "I recommend avoiding foods such as caffeine, tobacco, shellfish, niacin, red wine, pepper spices, and anything that triggers a flush."

Environmental factors such as sun exposure and stress will also aggravate redness, so make sunscreen your constant daytime companion throughout your treatment. Stress is also a factor. Do what you can to remain as calm, relaxed, and stress free as possible. (Check out chapters 7 and 8 for some ideas on what you can do to alleviate feelings of tension, anxiety, and pressure.)

Acne. When pimples pop up, treat them with appropriate medications, and then do what you can to camouflage them while they heal. "Acne is one of my patients' biggest issues," Dr. Wexler says. "I recommend salicylic acid over benzoyl peroxide because it's less drying, less irritating, and less likely to cause an allergic reaction."

When searching for products, Dr. Wexler says to look for those geared for adult skin. "They are usually synonymous with dryer skin, whereas many other acne products are formulated for oily skin."

"The key is to not overdry the skin," says Dr. Murad. "Use a mild cleanser during the day, and in the evening try an acne wash with salicylic acid to clean the pores gently. Apply a spot treatment with sulfur to the blemish as soon as the spot appears."

When it comes to covering up a blemish, our cosmetologists recommend a light touch.

"You can neutralize the red with a green- or yellow-based concealer," says Rick, "and then cover with foundation."

"With acne, I like to do the full makeup first," says Michele, "After that, if you find a spot is showing through, get one of those dry concealer pencils that have a little more yellow pigment in them and then just tap it on the pimple. With your finger tap a bit of foundation over that, then fix with powder."

"Go back to the color wheel," says Theresa. "If you want to hide red, select a concealer with a yellow or golden or beige undertone to it. Stipple it on, cover with a foundation or tinted moisturizer, or do the foundation first and then stipple on the concealer. The order is up to you, but if your acne gets severe, have your doctor take a look."

Uneven pigmentation.   Dark spots may appear on your skin, the result of sun exposure or heightened sensitivity to the sun or both due to chemotherapy. Regardless of the cause, there are products and treatments that can help reduce the appearance of spots and give your skin a more even tone throughout your treatment.

"Use SPF products every time you go outside," says Dr. Murad. "I've also found that applications of vitamin C will even the skin tone, while mineral makeups and camouflage-specific makeup from companies like *Cinema Secret* work great too."

"After sun protection, I find the best approach is to find a gentle peel designed for daily use," says Dr. Wexler. "I suggest trying it once a week, then twice a week, increasing as tolerated."

Dr. Wexler also recommends using brighteners and lighteners. "Look for products that contain hydrochinone; Haloxyl, which is a peptide that lightens the skin; and botanical brighteners like birch, bearberry, licorice, white tea, and green tea—as long as it says lightening, it will help. Just follow the label directions."

If the situation is extreme, Dr. Wexler says a visit to the dermatologist is in order.

"Machines called LED or white commission diode machines alternate at a certain wavelength to stimulate new collagen and elastic tissue, giving new life to damaged skin. Most dermatologists have them in their offices, and if their use is appropriate for your condition, they are readily available."

If an uneven complexion is bothering you, give yourself enough time to work out a camouflage routine.

"It can take some time, but if you're patient, you can use two foundations, one lighter and one darker, and stipple them together to even out your complexion," says Theresa.

Harvey agrees the best approach to hyperpigmentation is to camouflage until treatment is over. "If your sun protection and anti-inflammatory products are not taking care of the problem, then work with foundation, and also seek out products with vitamin C."

Rashes.   While they may be irritating or uncomfortable, rashes can also be a signal of an adverse reaction to your treatment.

"Your skin is the barometer of what is going on inside your body," Dr. Wexler says. "A rash is not a rash is not a rash, and if you're having a problem, you need to see your doctor."

Allergic reactions to chemotherapy are common, and the possibility that your rash represents such a situation cannot be ignored.

"If it looks like hives or insect bites, that's an emergency," Dr. Wexler says. "Call your doctor right away."

If you find you have a rash in the skin folds of your body (under the arms, under the breasts, in your groin area), that may be a fungal infection due to your suppressed immunity. Your doctor should look at it and will most likely prescribe an antifungal medication.

Your rash may be shingles. It could be a sign of some other type of infection. Regardless, if you find your skin is featuring bumps, your first, immediate call should be to your doctor, who will want to examine you and advise your next steps.

If it turns out the rash is just a minor skin irritation, Dr. Murad says to treat it with emollient creams.

"Stay away from highly preserved products," says Harvey. "Look at the ingredients list. You don't want formaldehyde or any sort of heavy preservative. The shorter the list of ingredients, the better the chance they won't irritate your already hypersensitized skin."

Sunburn-like pain. Sometimes, though your skin looks fine, it may hurt as if you've had too much sun exposure. This is likely just a side effect of your treatment, though it, too, may indicate an allergic reaction. As with a rash, if you're experiencing any pain or discomfort, tell your doctor. Once you're given the news that this isn't a serious issue, our dermatological experts have some advice for treating the condition.

"Sarna lotion or Pramosone lotion are topical, anti-itch, antineuralgia preparations that may offer relief," says Dr. Wexler.

"Applications of a soothing gel like Pramagel or Sarna

help," Dr. Murad says. "These are over-the-counter products that can be found in most pharmacies."

Neuropathy.   As their treatment progresses, some chemo girls suffer from neuropathy, which is a tingling and numbness of the hands that makes using tools such as makeup brushes difficult to impossible.

If you find yourself in this situation, our experts have some advice.

"Use creamy products instead of powders," says Anastasia, "and apply them with the tips of your fingers."

"People underestimate Q-tips," says Louis Philippe. "They're clean and they're disposable, and if you take the time to learn how to use them, they're great. You can also use smaller tools and sponges. Remember, it's mostly about blending. Use a light hand, blend your products in, and take it slowly."

"If you're really struggling with pencils and powders, eyebrows can be especially difficult," says Theresa. "In this situation, get a stencil, stick your finger in the powder, press it into the stencil, and color in the space. The stencil will make it easier, because you can go outside the lines."

Michele says fingers can do the work if your hands can't operate a brush. "Use the ring finger on either hand, or look in the drugstore for little applicators that can help your makeup session become a very easy process."

Excessive melanin.   Darker-skinned women sometimes suffer from excessive melanin production, which causes extreme color changes on the palms of the hands.

"It's important to know this so that if it happens, there's no need to panic," says Theresa. "Don't bleach it or use abrasives. It will take a bit of time, but once your chemo is over, this will go away."

Keeping your sunny side up. Be patient with yourself during this time of change. Believe in your absolute right to feel good about the way you look, and never lose your ability to transform.

"This is just a momentary passage of time," Michele reminds us. "I had a friend on chemo, and she looked very glamorous, with cheekbones like a 1940s movie star. She was so afraid of what was going to happen to her looks, yet in the end, it wasn't nearly as bad as she imagined. In fact, she actually looked quite good."

"A woman should not feel trivialized because she wants to maintain her appearance during illness," Dr. Wexler says. "No one wants to look sick, and a woman facing chemotherapy should continue to look her best, because looking healthy isn't vain, it's an important step toward feeling healthy."

Consider the whole package, says Louis Philippe. "It's not about lips or eyes, it's about balancing your look and projecting the type of person you are. Let your schedule help you make appropriate use of your makeup. During the day, when there's more light, use the same colors, but with less intensity, and if you're going out after dark, use full color."

"Makeup is all about accentuating the positive," Theresa says. "If you don't like your nose, play up your eyes. No hair? Then play up your lips. Chemo doesn't take away from who you are. It's all temporary, just a bump in the road. These conditions will go away once your treatment is over."

"There is no blanket approach to these problems," Michele says. "Take the time to find what works best for you. Don't think about what you looked like before you got sick, just deal with the now. It's only a moment in time. When it's over and you're feeling fine again, you'll be able to look back and say, 'Yeah, I did it.'"

A chemo girl is a woman who is strong; a fighter, determined to be well. Let your desire to triumph over illness radiate from within, and use your inner strength to empower yourself to look as good as you wish.

Don't avoid invitations or hide when the camera comes out. Enhance your overall well-being in whatever way works best for you, and never forget that in the not-so-distant future, when this is all in the past, you will indeed be able to say, "I did it."

To learn more about the information discussed in this chapter, please visit these websites:

www.lookgoodfeelbetter.org

www.murad.com

www.patriciawexlermd.com

www.skinsciencerb.com

www.bathandbodyworks.com

www.anastasia.net

www.micheleburke.com

www.elcompanies.com

www.physiciansformula.com

www.sephora.com

www.americanbeautycosmetics.com

www.kohls.com

www.biafine.orthoneutrogena.com/prescribinginfo.asp

www.cinemasecrets.com

CHAPTER 4

Chemo Style

THE SURVIVORS REMEMBER

Marybeth: With my weight gain, nothing fit me, so I took to wearing yoga pants, loose shirts, and baggy jeans. The funny thing is, I got so used to being in bigger clothes, it's now hard for me to wear anything that's formfitting or sexy; I just want to be comfy.

Chris: Because of my weight gain, I had to buy new clothes two sizes up. Just about everything I selected was black because it slims better than any other color and looks very stylish. But I was happy to be able to get back into my old clothes again. I missed them!

Laura: I always "dressed up" for chemo treatments and medical appointments. It made me feel better to look my best. Tops were a bit of a trick as my bilateral mastectomy left me with purple scars across the front of each breast. I became the trendsetter in layering and found a really cute thin strap tank that I wore under everything! I still wear just an elastic starter-style bra for fear of damaging the implants.

Patricia: I wore comfortable, classy flat shoes, pants with an elasticized waist, and button-down shirts. I think a designer who could come up with some tops with a high neckline would find a big market with mastectomy patients. We still want to look sexy!

Rosemarie: I didn't have much weight gain, so my pants were okay, but I mostly wore dresses or skirts to work and sweatpants at home. I wore exercise bras because they were more comfortable, and I found that button-down shirts or jackets with a zipper worked for me. I also wore a cross my sister gave me, not as much for religious reasons, as it just made me feel good to have it on.

The Side Effects

bloating	sallow skin
weight gain	ashy skin
weight loss	hyper-skin sensitivity

The Pearls

Once you have your hair and skin situations in hand, you may find that a key question regarding your outer beauty remains: What should I wear?

Because of side effects of your treatments, you may open your closet and not find clothes that will help you feel comfortable, stylish, and put together. Regardless of what sort of challenges your body is facing, our experts have tapped into their collective well of fashion know-how to give you the guidance you'll need. If it's important to you, you can continue to look as fashionable as you wish, no matter what the treatment may be doing to your weight, your skin, or your style.

When it comes to getting dressed, "You dictate what people will see when they look at you," says Francine DeMarco. "So the illusion you create with your clothes and accessories will draw the eye away from trouble spots. When you make the right choices, no one will have any idea you're concealing a flaw."

Fashion, like makeup, is the art of emphasis: draw the observer's eye where you want it to go, and no one will notice what you want to hide.

"Conceal, cover, and wear some things that will make you relax," says Betsey Johnson. "Concentrate on what's comfortable, because great style always reflects a sense of ease in your clothes."

WHAT'S GOING ON

There are a variety of reasons for your body to change its shape or size while undergoing chemotherapy. Steroids and other antinausea drugs can generate fat deposits from your arms to your thighs. Some drug combinations, rather than make you sick, cause an increase in appetite. Couple this with fatigue, which is perhaps the most common side effect of all cancer treatments, and you have a perfect recipe for putting on extra pounds.

You may not be adding fat to your frame. You may just be retaining water. And then there are the thousands of chemo girls who react in the opposite way to their treatment and get so thin their clothes hang off them, as if they were purchased for someone else.

Skin can react very quickly to the onslaught of chemo, becoming so sensitive that only the softest, most natural fabrics will feel comfortable. And as we discussed in chapter 3, you may find your complexion turning sallow if you're light skinned, turning ashy if you're dark, or looking just pale and washed out as treatment continues.

Dealing with these side effects is the price we pay to take the treatment that'll make us well. We don't have to lose our sense of fashion or self as we move toward health. We can still carry on our lives as they were before the diagnosis and look the way we want to look, regardless of where the treatment falls on the calendar. Our experts have provided a lot of solid advice to help you keep a working wardrobe together while you deal with this business of cancer, finish your therapy, and move on with the rest of your life.

What to Do

"Women instinctively know what looks good on them," Leah Berkowitz says. "The trick is to figure out how to cope with problems that come up so that you can go out feeling good about what you have on, and confident with the way you look."

"We're all stylists," Francine agrees. "We just don't realize that the tools we need to create our own signature style are probably right in our closets or just a shopping trip away."

Wearing clothes we like makes us feel happy and self-assured. Facing sudden changes to our face and figures can leave us lost as to how we're to camouflage what on our bodies we don't want people to see.

As with our makeup choices, we need to look at the whole picture and decide what still works, what about us remains a positive focal point, and then make the subtle adjustments to our wardrobe to make that feature pop.

"Yves Saint Laurent taught me that it's about the whole woman," says Louis Philippe DeMontpensier. "You must think about the entire image. When she walks into a room, people take in everything about her—her face, her hair, her clothes, and accessories. A balance of these things represents the entire picture."

Christine DeAngelo agrees. "It's all about balance and proportion," she says. "Play with different styles and cuts, get a feel for what is comfortable and looks good, and then go with it."

"Fashion is personal," says Betsey. "If you look in the mirror and what you have on makes you feel uplifted and positive, then you've done what you need to do."

According to Betsey, there are no real rules. "You can use whatever elements are out at the moment to add to your look, make it hip and cool. Don't worry about that as much as what psychologically makes you feel better.

"Make your clothes a celebration," she advises. "The message is really about how you feel. If you want to wear a turquoise turtleneck and a huge necklace when the designers are saying "Oh no, stick to black," remember that your true beauty is in your spirit. Just be true to your own personal preferences, and you will go out into the world very self-assured, very comfortable. That is where the confidence comes from—feeling good about yourself."

Laying the Foundation

Being at ease in your clothes is the paramount consideration right now. You don't want cuts that bind, fabrics that irritate, or styles that make you feel self-conscious about what you're going through. The very first garments you put on your body will have a direct effect on how relaxed and easy you feel for the rest of the day.

"The undergarments you choose are going to affect how your clothes fit you and how comfortable you'll be in them all day long," Francine says. "This isn't the time for lace and nylon—those fabrics will irritate. Instead, pick Pima or brushed cotton, anything that's going to feel good as soon as it brushes your skin."

Many chemo girls wear sports bras during treatment because they're supportive, soft, and available in fabrics that absorb or "wick away" excessive perspiration. Or you may want to try a jersey cotton camisole with a shelf bra.

"It's all personal choice," says Francine. "There are so many blends and weaves out now that are natural and breathable, especially with workout clothing. You can buy wonderful exercise pants and tops that move with you; they stretch and they give and they let you be as active as your body will allow."

Don't put on undergarments that make you aware of the fact that you have them on. A thong that makes you want to pick at your bottom, a bra that makes you feel trussed, and a fabric that scratches—these are items to put in the back of your drawer, at least for now.

"It's funny, because people tend to associate fashion with discomfort," Christine says. "You know, high heels and tight fits. But the truth is real fashion is about feeling good in your clothes, and unless they're comfortable, you're not going to project that sense of ease that good style always inspires in the wearer."

Chemo Style—It's in the Eyes . . .

Once your foundation garments have been chosen, look at yourself in a full-length mirror and decide what about you looks the same as ever, then pick out clothes that work around that still wonderful feature.

"When I dress people," Francine says, "I look at their eyes, because they are the one thing that never changes. I choose a hue that brings out the color of the eyes."

Betsey is a big fan of color. "I can't wear black, it's just too depressing for me," she says. "When it comes to color, pick any one that you want and that is going to make you feel good. If you're not sure, show a friend, and she'll tell you if it works."

"If it makes you come alive, you know you're on the right track," Francine says in agreement. "And you know, we may be darker in summer and paler in winter, but we tend to dress in a certain palate all year round. Why? Because we dress in the colors that bring out our eyes. Ask most women what their favorite color is and more times than not you'll find it's one that makes their eyes stand out."

Go to a boutique or department store, hold up various garments while looking in the mirror, find the hues that will enhance the color in your eyes, and then check in your closet and drawers to see what you already have that will do the job.

Continue to search for the best selections in your personal fashion palate. Once you're satisfied you've collected the ones that'll make you look your best, choose the styles that feel most comfortable when you've got them on.

. . . and the Size

How much you enjoy wearing an article of clothing has as much to do with how it hangs as how it looks. Proper fit ensures that you cover both criteria, as clothes that swim on you, pinch you, or make you look stuffed inside will simply not give you the style and silhouette you desire.

Once you've established your best color choices, you can concentrate on the matter of appropriate fit. While snug pants may be tolerable when you're well, the last thing a chemo girl needs is the feeling of being in something that's too small. Oversized shirts may generally look great on a girl, but when one is going through significant weight loss, oversized outfits spotlight the fact that the wearer's health is compromised.

Take a page from *Goldilocks*, and only go for the things that fit "just right."

"If you're in the store trying things on, sit down and see how the clothes feel," Christine says. "Do they cut into your stomach or thighs? If so, get the next size up."

"Some people think, 'Oh if I get the bigger size, I'll look bigger,'" she continues, "but it's really the opposite. If you're wearing a size that's too small and doesn't fit, you'll look too big for the clothes you have on."

Unless chemo has whittled your body down to serious thinness, a good rule of thumb is to err on the side of larger, Christine advises.

"If you have to hold your breath or lie down to zip your pants or your movement is restricted—you know, you can't take a full step because the thighs are too tight—then you need to move up a size or go for a different rise or cut. There are so many different options in slacks now, from skinny to relaxed, that the attention has to be on what gives you the best fit and look."

If your sleeves are too tight, or perhaps your shirt feels stretched across your back, revisit your closet, search your drawers, and find pieces that offer a little more room. You won't look or feel your best if you're squeezing into your clothes, and while we all want our favorite outfits to fit, during chemo this may be an elusive goal.

Once treatment is over, your body will most likely return to its former shape and size, so don't beat yourself up over a pair of jeans or a beloved sweater that is suddenly not fitting the way you like. Instead, find clothes that let you walk, sit, relax, and breathe easily. Choose fabrics that feel soft against your skin and styles that compliment your chemo-altered shape.

"It all breaks down to how it makes you feel," Betsey says. "If it's a style you want to try or a color you love, put it on, and as long as it fits and you like what you see, go ahead and wear it."

All About Proportions

"Healthy or not, we all have figure flaws we want to hide," Francine says. "Women often have hips that are wider than their shoulders, or a rounded belly, or thighs they find too big. As stylists, we build in the proportion nature hasn't provided, so that these irregularities become hidden."

For instance, if you're finding that treatment is causing some fluid retention in your thighs and making you look bottom heavy, a jacket or off the shoulder shirt will draw the eye upward, away from what you don't want people to see. Coupled with a pair of full cut, wide leg, or relaxed fit pants in a darker tone, a bright top helps even out your silhouette, slim your legs, and pull the gaze toward your face.

If a belly is your problem, consider pants that rise a bit higher, coupled with a longer, tunic-type top, a blousy tee, or a button-down shirt with a tailored shirttail that falls below your waistline. If your arms are not looking their best, consider blouses with fuller sleeves. If your hips are driving you batty, try wearing a shirt that falls below your bottom—or change things up completely and put on a dress.

"I'm a big fan of dresses," Leah says. "You can get jersey cotton dresses and wear them with cotton leggings. You can pick out a tent dress or an A-line. They are both very comfortable."

Dresses are a favorite choice for Christine too. "A-lines are great, and so are full skirts. These cuts always work because you don't really know what's going on underneath them."

Create a sense of balance with your shape, and pull the gaze away from what you don't like and toward something you're happy with.

"Use lighter shades where you want the eye to travel, and darker shades on the areas you're not as comfortable with," Betsey says. "Don't separate yourself from looking at fashion magazines. If it's something you enjoy, don't deny yourself that pleasure. I think it's really important and inspiring to keep up with what's going on because that way you don't have to feel life has changed so radically. You can still be curious about what's happening, be interested in what's new and cool, and get whatever ideas will suit the way your body is right now."

In the Eye of the Beholder

As Academy Award–winning makeup artist Michele Burke said in chapter 3, when people look at you, their eyes will generally focus on one point of your face or body. Whether it's your lips, your neck, or your hands, the power to decide where you want that eye to land is under your control.

"Let's say you're not happy with your middle right now,"

Francine says. "You can't slim yourself down in time for lunch, but you can direct where you want people to look so that a bloated waistline or a flabby belly is essentially invisible."

"Wear an open-toed shoe with bright toenail polish," she advises. "Dress in a monotone that compliments your eye color and accessorize with a contrasting scarf and bag. Wear earrings that are noticeable under your wig, and show a little bit of skin, maybe at your neck, or your collar bone, or, if you have it, décolletage. The eye will always go where skin is showing, and it will naturally drift from one of your chosen focal points to another, and absolutely no one will notice your middle."

That is the magic of illusion and distraction. Imagine going out one afternoon to meet a friend for lunch, dressed as Francine describes. A diner sitting across the restaurant, distracted by your shoes, your skin, and your fashion contrasts will admire your pedicure, your bag, or your scarf. Those sitting at your table will appreciate your earrings, or the way your eye color pops and sparkles. No one will perceive that your torso is not as fit or slender or shapely as you might wish it to be.

You don't have to go out and spend a lot of money on new things. As long as the clothes you have fit, it's really just a matter of deciding which items work best on your body now. If you find that you do need a wardrobe shopping trip to accommodate your changing dimensions, do an inventory of what you already have first so that you don't end up buying things you don't really need.

It's entirely possible that your closet and jewelry box contain most of what you'll need to get through chemo in comfort and style. If you just add a few additional staples, you'll be able to round out your options for a variety of looks.

Consider adding a full skirt; some soft, billowy shirts; wide-legged pants; or an A-line dress to your wardrobe to create a base from which you can build a signature style. You can find most of these items in stores ranging from discount to designer. Then pick out a trendy bit of costume jewelry, find a pair of sleek flat shoes, or don a funky hat, and suddenly the ordinary becomes exotic. People won't be preoccupied with how you're feeling—instead they'll be pleased with how well you look.

"Think of Audrey Hepburn in *Breakfast at Tiffany's*," Francine says. "So many books and articles about her say she didn't like her figure at all. But she was considered an international beauty. Why? Well remember her little black dress? It wasn't exactly revolutionary. But add the hat, the sunglasses, and the gloves—and suddenly she's a woman like no other. She's an icon. No one cared about her skinny little body or her long neck or any of the things she supposedly didn't find attractive about herself. They were too mesmerized by the big picture. With just a few great wardrobe choices she created an image the fashion world will never forget."

All About Accessories

When it comes to creating a totally together outfit, what is it that designers, stylists, and fashion mavens absolutely can't live without?

Accessories!

From Coco Chanel's pearls to the famous dark glasses sported by Jackie Onassis, accessories have the power to take the ordinary and make it extraordinary.

"I love accessories," Leah says. "They're so much fun to buy and wear, and a few changes can make the same outfit look different every day."

When considering options, "Go for dangling earrings," Leah advises, "or a long chain with a charm that falls to the middle of your torso. These things will elongate you, make you look pretty and feminine and will take attention away from whatever it is you don't want to highlight.

"Or just treat yourself to a great bag or great shoes," she says. "They always work, they finish a look, and they're lots of fun to wear."

Francine reminds us of some of the last century's larger-than-life fashionistas and the accessories that helped create their image: "Women like Princess Diana, Jackie O, Grace Kelly, and Marilyn Monroe all knew that a well-chosen accessory would frame their public persona. A scarf, a ring, a hat—they found the items that worked for them. Their selections were so successful, they created cottage industries for their look. People flocked to stores to emulate these styles, and the things they chose to wear twenty or fifty years ago still work today."

What sort of accessories should you consider when you want to create a stylish presentation during treatment? It really comes down to just a few items—a fabulous bag, some flat shoes, maybe a hat, a couple of scarves, and, most importantly, the right jewelry.

"Jewelry and clothing should reflect purity to symbolize the healing power of nature and spirit," says Robert Lee Morris. "When jewelry can act like a worry stone, or a rosary, it causes the wearer to participate in the spirit of the piece, and the repetitive action of touching and stroking helps calm the nerves."

Robert's work conveys of sense of well-being and comfort to the wearer. His philosophy is to work with metal, not stones or other precious commodities. "When you're going through any kind of personal crisis, you want to wear jewelry that imparts a sensual, sculptural experience," he says. "It shouldn't be about bling right now, but about tranquility. You want pieces that are smooth to the touch, inviting the wearer to caress, and perhaps commune with, the warm earthiness of the piece."

When deciding which pieces to select, Leah offers one caution, "I wouldn't suggest chokers, short strands, anything tight around the neck." That will just bring attention to your skin tone, your missing hair, or anything else about your face you're not thrilled with. Instead, try a long gold or a soft sheen necklace that draws the focal point away from your head and toward your heart."

"Wearing symbols of beautiful objects, ancient symbols of love, life, hope, and peace, is inspirational," says Robert. "Jewelry for women in crisis should be therapeutic and comforting. Think of it as a pet or a close friend. You don't want anything over the top right now. I would suggest warm bronze, fragrant sandalwood—these natural products of the earth will do a lot to raise your self-esteem and give you a feeling of peace."

Options are available at every price point.

"Costume jewelry has come so far, you can always find something to make you happy without breaking the bank," Francine says. "I think it's perfectly reasonable to treat yourself to something special right now, something that you can wear throughout your chemo that is going to make you feel good whenever you have it on."

The choices, Francine says, are vast. "A ring or a bangle or a special charm on a chain—whatever it is that appeals to you, you can admire it even as you're wearing it and enjoy the experience of having this special piece as a salute for all you're enduring."

Leah says if she were shopping for her "must have" accessory, "I'd go out and get myself a fantastic bag. It's just so much fun to go bag shopping. There are so many choices, and they're really gorgeous. It's not about how it fits or whether it's comfortable, it's just about the fact that you love it and are excited to carry it."

Leah says once you have a great bag, you'll be more likely to want to go out so that you can show it off.

"I think it's important for chemo patients to look good when they leave the house," she says. "Don't go to the doctor in crummy old jeans and a faded sweatshirt because that just feeds into the concept that you're sick and that your body isn't in the place you want it to be.

"Fix yourself up and be excited about the way you look," Leah advises. "Put on pretty dangling earrings and classy comfortable shoes and carry a fabulous bag. If you live in jeans, pick out a pair of black or gray instead of the standard blue and throw on a soft, cotton T-shirt, and you're there—you look like a celebrity."

Cottoning to Your Clothes

In the quest for comfort, our experts agree that cotton reigns supreme. It's soft, it wears and washes well, it breathes and absorbs perspiration, and it's completely natural.

"I can't wear anything but cotton," says Betsey. "As much as I love cashmere and linen and silk and all that, they're too hot and scratchy for me."

"Jersey cotton, overwashed cotton, Pima cotton—there are so many choices with this fabric," Leah says. "No matter where you shop, you will be able to find cotton garments that have the cut and the style and the color you want. Just pick out whatever feels good to the touch."

Christine adds that silk, linen, and gauzy materials may be worth a try. "Always wear natural fibers, but choose the more breathable fabrics. Wool may be natural, but it's just too irritating to the skin. A soft silk sweater will keep you just as warm in the winter, and it won't cause you to break out in a rash.

"In the warmer weather," she continues, "if you have a soft linen or gauze or maybe a knit silk you want to try, just hold it against your skin to see how you feel. If it's light and airy, and you don't get a reaction, itching or any kind of irritation, and you like the way it looks, then wear it."

Francine says when it comes to making a chemo-style

decision, the answer may be as easy as pajamas: "Rather than spend a lot of time trying to work out all these different style ideas, you could just live in loungewear," she says. "I can't tell you how many times I've gone to someone's house in what are actually a nightshirt and pants, and the girls I'm visiting have flipped over my fabulous clothes!"

Francine says if your goal is to be chic and comfortable all the time, head to the loungewear department of your favorite store and let loose. "They've come so far in design, there are dozens of choices, from jersey cotton to brushed velvet to knit silk. They are so comfortable and stylish and affordable, you can wear them every day. With one outfit, you're comfortable, stylish, fabulous, and you're still in your pajamas! It's like a fashion *grand slam!*"

Hide and No One Will Seek

Each of the side effects that may have an impact on your body shape offers its own set of challenges. While our great hope is that you never need any of the following information, if it turns out that chemo is causing a reaction you want to camouflage, our experts have provided these specific tips to help you create the illusion that hides whatever you are not thrilled with. You can continue to face the world looking the way you want until the day when you are free and clear of chemo and can put this whole experience behind you.

Use the suggestions that follow to figure out how to dress

when your body isn't behaving. While you may have to add some items to your closet, don't redo your wardrobe. What is happening to you is temporary. These side effects will end when treatment does. You'll bounce back, you will go on with your life, and you won't need many of the things that right now seem essential.

Be kind to yourself. When you look in the mirror, try to appreciate everything that you're doing to get through this experience. Make it a point to admire your own strength and courage. Even if you're not thrilled with the way you look, give a silent shout out to the spirit inside you that keeps fighting.

Our experts offer their take on how to deal with specific body challenges that are making it harder for your wardrobe to work. When you consider your clothes each morning, you don't need to feel lost or confused. You'll be excited about what you're going to wear and how nice it's going to make you look.

Excessive Thinness

Contrary to the Duchess of Windsor's famous belief about riches and slimness, every chemo girl who has lost a lot of weight during treatment knows that while you may indeed never be too rich, you can, in fact, be too thin. When your body is losing a lot of its lean body mass due to treatment, it's no healthier, and no more fashionable, than trying to deal with unwanted pounds.

But there are things you can do to make the most of

your narrower silhouette and at the same time enjoy some good fashion fun.

"Layering is always a great option," Christine says. "A vest over a tank top and then maybe a little jacket over that will add some bulk."

"You can also try drapes and ruched styles like cowl necks, wrapped skirts, and dresses," she continues. "These fabrics will make you look more rounded."

"You don't want to look like you're swimming in your clothes," Leah says, "so I would say a proper fit is paramount. Try skinny jeans with a T-shirt and a vest, and cover up your chest or shoulders if they're becoming very bony.

"Thin arms and legs work with almost any style," Leah says, "so choose outfits that are appropriate for your new shape.

"If your clothes are the right size, you'll just look like you're a thin woman, and there's nothing wrong with that. Don't go for things that swallow you up, as that will just draw attention to your weight loss. Concentrate on layering and stay away from the baggy, oversized look until you return to your regular size."

While black may be the perfect shade for fashion leaders, this is no time to dress from head to toe in the color known for its slimming prowess.

"If you're very thin, go for colors," says Betsey. "Vibrant colors will liven you up. You can wear a T-shirt or a blouse and then a bulky sweater over it and you'll look really hip and bright. That will definitely elevate your mood."

Dresses will do wonders for whatever wardrobe problems ail you.

"The wrap dress is a classic," Francine says, "and it will do wonders for a figure that is very thin."

"Dresses are really the best form of clothing because they are the ultimate disguise," she adds. "Nobody can see if your weight is on the way up or on the way down, and they create a unified look that's a great base to work from."

Stay away from very tight clothes.

"Tightness will just emphasize how slender you've become," says Francine. "Make sure your clothes fit well, but stay away from snug styles. They won't compliment your figure as much as draw attention to a thinness that is a direct result of being sick."

Altered Skin Tone

Just as your makeup choices may have to adjust to a yellowish or ashy tone to your skin, the clothes you wear will make this condition either more obvious or much less noticeable.

"Remember what I said about dressing for your eyes?" Francine asks. "This is a great example of why that is so important. If you're working with shades that bring out your eye color it won't really matter what your skin tone has become—you'll still look good."

"If you're sallow, I would stick with warmer tones," Christine says, "because if you try to wear any of the cool colors, you're going to be opposing what's going on with your skin and calling attention to it."

"I would avoid yellow and green and brown," Leah says

about women with sallow skin. "They'll just make your skin color look more obvious."

Francine agrees. "You want to stay away from stark white and acid yellow, or what I call the 7-Up colors," she says. "Anything lemon or lime is going to be a mistake for a woman with sallow skin."

If you're ashy, try wearing brighter, cooler colors.

"If your skin is brown or chocolate or black, any color is going to look good on you," Leah says. "I would say if you start to look a little gray, or maybe you have some hyperpigmentation going on, try turquoise or coral or another vibrant shade. But I wouldn't wear yellow. That's not the best choice right now."

Christine agrees. "I think the cool tones are what you need," she says. "Blue, purple, and berry are all good choices. I wouldn't wear black or gray or anything that is close to the color of your skin, because then the contrast is right there and it's easy to see something about your natural color is off."

If you're pale or just not looking as rosy as you'd like, Francine says go back to her edict: dress for the eyes.

"If you dress in a way that makes their color sparkle, that's where people will look," she says. "That's where your real beauty is, anyway. That's where your soul shines."

The Finishing Touches—Hats and Scarves

For every woman who loves a hat, there is at least one more who has never worn a chapeau any more elegant than a baseball cap or hood.

During chemotherapy, hats can be invaluable wardrobe assets. Consider the appeal: they keep the sun away from our skin. They cover our heads, protecting our tender scalp and shielding the casual observer from seeing whatever may be going on with our hair, from getting thin to missing to growing back. They also pull the eye away from the body, which our experts encourage. And they're fun.

"You can get a funky hat and a bandana," Leah says. "And if you really don't want to wear the wig one day, tie the scarf around your forehead, kind of low over the eyebrows, and then let some extra fabric fall down your back. Put a hat over that and you've got a great look."

And if you're not comfortable wearing a wide-brimmed affair?

"Hats are very personal," Francine says. "A lot of women don't feel at ease in them because people look at you when you have one on. That's not a feeling all women like, especially when they're sick and not feeling great about the way they look."

She recommends looking through magazines to see what the celebrities are wearing, and then heading out to whereever it is you like to shop best. Chances are they have something similar to what you've liked.

"Hats and scarves can take a good outfit and make it spectacular," Francine says. "You can be sick and still be spectacular if you feel like it."

She maintains that the benefits of wearing a hat, especially if you're getting treatment in the summer, should inspire at least one shopping trip in search of the perfect head cover.

"You can go to Henri Bendel or TJ Maxx or any store in between. You'll find so many choices, I really think you'll find one that works for you. Bring a friend and make it a little adventure, like a scavenger hunt to find another piece of your chemo armor."

While you're in the hat department, take a walk over to see what scarves may strike your fancy.

"Scarves are like hats," Francine says. "They make you look finished and completely put together."

"If you find some soft jersey cotton scarves in a bunch of colors and you have a few monotone foundations that fit and are comfortable, you really have all you need to look very stylish every day," she says.

When shopping for scarves, Leah says to narrow your choices to those that are light and soft. "They should be cotton, of course, the softest ones you can find. When you get home, wash them a bunch of times. If they have some fringe you can let flow from behind, that looks so pretty and feminine. Wear a straw fedora with some fringe coming down the back and you're perfect.

"Don't bother with the smaller sizes," she advises. "Get the large kind that are intended for your neck, the ones that have a lot of extra fabric after you've tied them," Leah advises. "That's what makes wearing them fun—playing with the extra once your head is covered."

Marilyn Monroe in the Park

Now that you have some basic concepts of how to make the most of your wardrobe during treatment, remember that when it comes to how you're perceived, your power isn't in your clothes or your makeup. It's in you.

"I once read a story about Marilyn Monroe," Francine says. "She supposedly was not comfortable in her own skin. She was being interviewed by a reporter in Central Park, and she had on dark sunglasses and a kerchief and had her image completely pulled in. At one point the reporter said to her, 'It's astonishing that we're here, in the middle of Central Park and nobody recognizes you.' And Marilyn replied, 'That's because I don't have "her" out there.' She was well aware of her power. To prove her point, she started walking her famous walk, and smiling, and laughing, and projecting her incomparable image. Within moments, they were mobbed by fans."

"What I love about this story is that whatever style Marilyn had didn't come from what she was wearing," Francine says. "It was inside her. She turned it on."

We all have the ability to do what Marilyn did. The way we project ourselves determines how people see us. When it comes to getting dressed when we're undergoing chemotherapy, the key is to pick out whatever is comfortable and relaxing and makes us feel good, and then go out into the world with confidence.

Projecting your inner beauty, your spirit, and your radiance will do more to enhance your look than anything you could possibly put on. Do whatever you wish to look as good as you can. The guiding fashion principle is to hide, distract, and pull attention away from trouble spots and to seek, encourage, and create an attractive focal point with your clothes and accessories.

Cast yourself as the director of your image and make yourself your very own star. Wear things that inspire tranquility and comfort, and let your own amazing life force be the power that ensures your beauty.

If you use your indomitable spirit as your essential foundation, no matter what you wear will be more than fashionable—it will be fabulous—and you will move through your chemo confident in yourself, at ease with your situation, and in control of your image.

You'll be Marilyn Monroe in the park.

CHAPTER 5

The Business of You

THE SURVIVORS REMEMBER

Marybeth: I woke up one night with a dreadful head pain that grew worse as the hours went on. Over-the-counter medications did nothing. When morning came, my husband called my oncologist, who confirmed that a rare side effect of my chemo was migraine headaches. We got a prescription, and within a few hours I was fine. After that, I made it my business to call the doctor's office whenever something hurt. They always found a way to make the pain go away.

Laura: My nails peeled and broke and turned a weird color. I was very careful about germs; my middle child was in kindergarten and I avoided his school for most of the year!

Rosemarie: My hips and legs ached and it was hard to sleep without a pillow between my legs. But once treatment ended, that was it. Everything went away.

The Side Effects

bone pain	insomnia
muscle aches	fatigue
constipation	headaches
diarrhea	numbness/neuropathy
drowsiness	nausea

The Pearls

Beauty is more than the condition of your hair and skin. If your body is not functioning properly, all the style in the world won't hide the physical manifestations of the inner struggles you face.

When you're undergoing chemotherapy, a host of body-altering side effects come into play. While a lovely wig or well-applied foundation will help camouflage some of these issues, looking good is predicated on feeling good. The best way to achieve this during cancer treatment is to take care of your body. Listen to what it needs and supply what it requires, and the radiance of inner strength and balance will shine through.

More than any previous time in your life, you are going to need help to get through the logistics of treatment with the least amount of stress possible. The best way to ensure that you accomplish chemo with strength and calm is to do what may seem unimaginable in your healthy, everyday life—ask for help.

"Women have a hard time being receivers," says cancer and mastectomy massage specialist Cheryl Chapman. "We're trained to be caregivers, but this is the time where you have to indulge yourself. As much as you can, you have to be selfish."

If you're willing to open up about how someone can be of assistance, you'll find a lot of helping hands waiting to be called on. It's support you'll need—for transportation to and from infusions, for babysitting children if you have them, and for meals, grocery shopping, and trips to the drugstore. By enlisting others to do these things for you, you'll lighten your load, get more accomplished, and connect with those in your life and community who really want to be there for you. Taking hold of the hands offering assistance creates a winning situation for everyone who knows you.

"Don't be afraid to ask for the help you need," say the nurses at the Princeton Medical Group (PMG). "Take advantage of whatever help is offered. Let people drive for you or cook for you or run errands for you. Bring someone you trust to your doctor consultations so they can take notes and give you their sense of the fit between you and the potential caregiver.

"This is one time in your life," the nurses say, "where you'll find you really can't expect to do it all alone."

What's Going On

No matter how busy your world was before cancer, once the diagnosis is confirmed, your to-do list increases exponentially. A whirlwind of decisions must be made, and all very quickly. Do you need a surgeon, or will chemotherapy address the malignancy? Is radiation in the cards? Do you want to include alternative therapies in your treatment? Where are the best doctors in your geographic area for the type of cancer you have? Which practitioners make you feel the most at ease? Who comes with the best recommendations? What procedures, practices, doctors, and hospitals are covered by your insurance?

You must answer all these questions in a timely manner to expedite your cancer care with comfort and success.

"The patient must find an oncologist she identifies with, who she feels comfortable with, who she can ask questions of," says cancer survivor Dr. Leonard Wright. "She has to be able to have an open dialog. This is a team, a partnership, and the patient must be a fully active participant in the process."

In 1989, Dr. Wright was diagnosed with a brain tumor. Now the director of the Wege Institute for Mind, Body and Spirit at the Lack's Cancer Center in Grand Rapids, Michigan, he understands on an intimate level how important these early decisions about treatment will be.

"I contacted surgical oncologists all over the country and Canada," he remembers. "The *only* one who suggested he could remove the tumor surgically was my hometown neurosurgeon. Every other doctor said they wouldn't touch it because it was too close to the motor centers. So if I'd just listened to the first opinion I received and hadn't done the research, it's not likely I would've been able to practice medicine. I may not have even survived."

The right doctors—those who understand your condition, who have direct experience treating it, and with whom you feel a bond—are integral to your journey back

to wellness. Finding them takes time, patience, and per-severance.

"It's so important to get second opinions," says Dr. Wright. "Learn as much as you can about your condition. No matter where you live, get to your area's major medical center. It's worth the investment of time and energy to see someone at a Johns Hopkins or Memorial Sloan Kettering or M. D. Anderson because these people are doing the cutting-edge research that could make all the difference in your care."

Selecting Your Medical Team

To begin researching your options, do an Internet search of your particular cancer. Follow the links you've found to learn more about what you're facing. Put out the word through your local grapevine to discover who has been through a similar health crisis. Find out where they were treated and by whom. If your life doesn't include anyone who has either survived cancer or knows someone else who has, organizations such as Gilda's Club, Y-Me, The American Cancer Society, and others can provide some leads on where to turn.

Libraries often have computers. If your home or office doesn't offer online capabilities, go to a local branch and ask a staff member to set you up so that you can access the Web. Once you're there, type the words "cancer support groups" in the search bar, add your locality or state to the entry (i.e., cancer support groups, New York City), and see what organizations exist in your area. Social services are another great resource for information and direction. You

can contact churches, synagogues, mosques, community centers, and local hospitals for recommendations on doctors, services, and resources to utilize.

When collecting information online, Dr. Wright urges caution. "It's not all peer reviewed," he warns. "It's a blessing, in that we can learn a lot about what we're facing, but a curse in that we can't be sure if what we're reading is dependable, accurate information."

Use the Web to get basic information about surgical and treatment options. Take what you learn online, write down all the questions you have, and use these notes to interview doctors. Make informed decisions about the kind of care you want to receive as well as whom you choose to provide you with that care.

Once you locate the professionals you want to consider for your medical team, make a consultation appointment. Bring the films from X-rays, MRIs, and scans that identified your cancer; any doctor, lab, or pathology reports you've received; and a synopsis of the information and research you've done.

"Face-to-face meetings are wonderful because you'll know from being in the doctor's presence whether this person fits your style," says Dr. Wright. "It's crucial to your healing for you to be comfortable with your medical team. Ask all your questions and gauge how the doctors respond."

When you meet with various doctors, which strike you as being open minded? Who treats you with interest, courtesy, and sympathy? How many have hands-on experience with your specific condition? Whose treatment recommendations are in sync with what you've learned on your own

or heard about from other medical professionals? Do any of the doctors suggest approaches that are considered radical, trial, or outside the norm? On what data are they basing these recommendations?

Moving further into the area of an actual relationship with these providers, ask yourself how comfortable the doctor makes you feel? How much confidence is inspired as a result of your meeting? Is the doctor patient and kind? Is his or her personality a match for yours? Do you have a sense of trust in their ability to treat you? Do you feel as if you can establish a connection with this person? If you answered yes to these questions and their professional credentials are in order, you've found a health-care provider who can be a member of your team.

If you find during the visit or in follow-up contact you're not getting the answers you seek or if you don't feel simpatico with this person, cross that name off your list and move on to the next physician. The nature of this relationship is so personal, intimate, and immediate, it's crucial for you to choose only those practitioners who inspire your deepest trust, confidence, and respect.

Considering how busy most people are in their daily lives and how small the window of opportunity is to pursue all these options while still reeling from the news of a diagnosis, taking the time you need to conduct these one-on-one meetings may seem like a huge obstacle. Set all the other priorities of your life aside for the moment and concentrate on assembling the medical personnel necessary to become well. If you find that you simply can't do it—or do it all—now is the time to let go of pride and independence and reach out for the support of your community, your family, and your friends.

You + Your Oncology Team = BFF

The closest medical relationship you build around your cancer care will be with your oncology team.

This group includes your doctor, the doctor's support staff, and the oncology nurses who will administer the prescribed chemotherapy to you. Depending on the medical practice you have chosen to provide your treatment and your insurance coverage, your team may also include nutritionists, massage therapists, psycho-oncologists, fitness professionals, and spiritual advisers.

No matter how many people are involved in your care, clear, immediate, and direct communication of whatever needs, questions, experiences, or symptoms you're presenting is crucial to the quality and success of your treatment.

"An open dialog is essential," says Dr. Wright. "Patients must tell their oncologist everything that they are taking and everything that they are feeling, and they must ask any and all questions they have over the course of their treatment. The only way the doctor can effectively help you is if all the information is on the table."

If you've heard that a certain herb works wonders against cancer, ask your oncologist about it, but don't actually take it unless you're given the green light. Your doctor may tell you that its healing potential is not proven. You may learn that ingesting this herb could create a severe reaction if taken in conjunction with the chemo drugs you're receiving. It could render your chemo ineffective.

"So many people don't understand that herbs can be just as powerful as drugs," says eastern medical doctor Sandy Canzone. "It's not wise to put anything you don't fully understand into your body without professional oversight. You can't just read a list of herbs that treat cancer and start taking some. You don't know how they're going to react with chemotherapy drugs."

Inform your team of any physical changes you are experiencing while undergoing chemo, such as insomnia, heartburn, rashes, aches, or pains. If something seems off about the way you feel and you can't quite figure out what it is, get this information to your doctor.

An effective oncology team will accept your call gladly, provide you with the answers you seek, and follow up to ensure that whatever you are inquiring about is addressed. They will use this dialogue to help advance your care. The more informative you are about your experience, the better they will be to help you manage your treatment.

Oncology nurses are on the front lines of intervention. When selecting your team, pay particular attention to these professionals. To a large degree, your welfare depends on their care. When interviewing oncologists, visit their infusion room and talk with the nurses on staff.

"They should be friendly and doting and make their patients feel safe and cared for at all times," say the oncology nurses at PMG. "They should offer a direct phone line so that the patient can contact them without delay should there be a question or concern."

"The emphasis must be on respectful, helpful, healing medicine," Dr. Canzone says. "I'm an Eastern medical doctor, but it's really traditional medicine I'm practicing. I treat each patient as an individual. I listen to their needs and issues. I find out what the family makeup is, what the job situation is, what is happening in their minds, what their spiritual connections are, and what gives them nourishment.

"This once was the standard way of practicing all medicine," she continues, "but insurance procedures and mounting financial pressures have made spending the amount of time and energy necessary to create that one-on-one space with each patient much harder for doctors. In treating cancer, however, it's really important for all the chaos of diagnosis to be put in order by a team of practitioners who will honor each patient's individuality and situation."

Your medical team should recognize you as a person and not just another patient. They should be committed to getting to the root causes of what may ail you during your cancer journey. This will help you relax about the treatment process. You'll have faith and confidence in their ability, their attention, and care.

"So many people want to treat the symptom, but a good doctor will go deeper to find the reason behind the ache, or the insomnia, or whatever is wrong," says New York chiropractor and nutritionist Dr. Joann Weinrib. "I think it's dangerous to play with symptoms. I believe it's important to identify the why of the situation, not just the what, and work to alleviate what is happening by treating the reasons behind whatever is presented."

You've every right, and every reason, to contact your doctors whenever a symptom or need presents itself. You shouldn't ever feel like querying your doctor about an issue is equal to being difficult, or needy, or bothersome. Your doctor is never too busy to help you. The administrative staff will always have the time to take your call. Don't take a wait-and-see approach to unusual symptoms. If something doesn't seem right, your job is to let your doctors know. Until you do, they'll have no idea you're in need.

We all want to be good patients, and as women, most of us aim to please. Talk to your doctors and nurses about what's going on with your body, your family, and your emotions. Follow the directions you've been given, take your medications as prescribed, and convey information in a timely manner to those who need to hear it. This is the foundation for a healthy, positive relationship with your caregivers.

Chemo Time!

Once all your medical team decisions have been made and your treatment strategy established, it's time to receive the drugs that'll eliminate your malignancy.

The process of receiving chemotherapy is fairly simple. Depending on the type of cancer you've got, the drugs your doctor prescribes, and your insurance coverage, your chemotherapy will be administered either at home, a doctor's office, a clinic, the outpatient department at a hospital or as an admitted patient in a hospital. The most common way to receive the drugs is intravenously, as an outpatient.

Treatment schedules vary according to the individual's cancer, treatment goals, the drugs being used and the way your body responds to them. Chemo is administered in cycles, alternating between infusions and periods of rest that allow your body to recover and build healthy new cells. You may receive chemo every day, once a week, once every couple of weeks, or once a month.

Before your first infusion, your doctor should spend some time educating you about what to expect and what you must do to be in the best shape to receive your chemo. You will receive prescriptions for medications to take either before the treatment or after the infusion is completed. The oncologist will also give you a list of "normal" reactions, and those that should cause concern. The process of receiving your medications will be reviewed so that you understand what is about to take place.

"Take a tour of the infusion room and meet the nurses before your first day of chemo," suggest the PMG nurses. "You'll feel comfortable and relaxed about the surroundings, and recognize the staff that will be working with you."

Your doctor may prescribe an optional antianxiety medication for you to take before you arrive. While you may not have taken such medications before, your goal must be to do whatever it takes to get through it. If you find yourself tense and worried, take the prescribed medication.

"Sedatives will take away some of the angst associated with receiving chemo," say the PMG nurses. "At the beginning, when you don't really know what's going to happen, they can alleviate fear. Later on, they can just make the whole experience a little easier to deal with."

The nurses have additional advice to help you prepare for receiving treatment.

- Drink a lot of water throughout your treatment.

- Avoid dehydrating caffeinated beverages. The objective is to give your body maximum hydration.

- Bring a sweater with you because sometimes the rooms can be cold or the medications you receive will make you feel chilled.

- Tell the nurses if you have got a medical problem such as diabetes or high or low blood pressure. Even if you have already told the oncologist, repeat these things to the oncology nurses so they are aware of your condition.

Once you arrive in the room, the routine for chemo is pretty well set.

"A needle will be inserted into a vein, or a port if your doctor has prescribed one," explain the PMG nurses. "You can ask the nurse to freeze the skin at the insertion point if you're afraid of that initial prick. Once that needle is in place, the patient should feel nothing."

Infusion usually begins with some premedication administered via the IV, typically hydration and antinausea agents. You may feel a little light-headed or sleepy as these make their way into your system.

"Tell the nurse whatever you're feeling," the PMG nurses

say, "especially if you find yourself short of breath, tight in the chest, or if the area around the needle is burning."

Don't be shy around your nurses. Talk to them. They will be better able to take care of you.

While it's perfectly fine to eat or drink while receiving your chemo, keep in mind some simple courtesies when in the infusion room.

- Make sure that any foods you bring do not leave a strong odor, as it may upset other patients in the room.

- Avoid wearing perfume or cologne to your treatment because the sense of smell during chemo can be altered, and the scent you've applied could nauseate another patient.

- Limit your infusion-room company to one guest. It can be overwhelming to have too many people in the infusion room.

- Speak to your guest in a quiet voice.

- Bring a book, a magazine, or some headphones to listen to music if you are alone during infusion.

- Turn your cell phone off.

- Leave children with a caregiver. There is no one in the infusion room to care for them.

When your IV is completed, you'll be asked to sit for a bit to make sure you're not dizzy or out of sorts. When you're cleared to leave, you'll need a ride home. Once you get there, take it easy. Give your body a chance to adjust to the onslaught of anticancer chemicals now coursing through you.

"Some people feel the effects of their treatment right away, while others may take a day or two to react," say the nurses. "You'll want to reveal any and all concerns to your doctor. Postinfusion symptoms like fever, rash, diarrhea, or headaches are very common, but don't let that stop you from calling if you feel something isn't right. Use the direct phone line to your oncology nurses. Once they hear what's going on, they'll let you know what if anything you need to do."

Soothing What Ails You

After the infusion, your body will begin to react to the chemicals you've received. Some side effects, such as nausea or headaches, may occur immediately. Others, such as fatigue, may appear months later. While no one enjoys these ailments, there are many pathways to relief.

It is basically impossible to go through chemo unfazed by the drugs in your veins. Somewhere along the way, you will experience some difficulties. When you do, our experts suggest trying these solutions to help alleviate whatever ails you.

Bone/Muscle Aches and Pain

It's entirely possible that you may pull a muscle or develop a body pain during chemo that has nothing to do with your treatment. Don't assume that an ache or pain is unrelated. Don't brush it off. Find the root cause of the problem so that appropriate measures can be taken.

"Oftentimes patients come to me with symptoms that they don't realize are side effects of chemotherapy," says orthopedic surgeon Dr. Brian Torpey. "Pain, aches, stiffness in the joints, arthritis can all be the result of chemotherapy exposure."

As an orthopedic surgeon, Dr. Torpey often sees patients complaining of an ailment only to discover during their consultation that they're undergoing cancer treatment.

"If someone comes to me and they're experiencing arm pain, for example, I might be thinking they need physical therapy," he says. "Once I learn that they're undergoing chemo, that significantly changes how I process the information.

"It's important that patients be very clear when they discuss their pain and discomfort symptoms with their oncologists," Dr. Torpey continues. "We must make sure these symptoms aren't indicating the cancer presenting itself via metastasis. Regardless of what specialty the doctor practices, when it comes to cancer treatment and patient health, all of a patient's physicians need to be on the same page."

On hearing that you are having aches or pain in your bones, your oncologist will send you for scans to make sure the disease has not spread. Once you know metastasis is not to blame for your symptoms, you may begin a course of treatment.

"It's important for doctors to tease out why someone is hurting and establish an accurate diagnosis," says internationally renowned pain specialist Dr. Peter Staats. "Commonly the small fibers of the nerve have been damaged by chemotherapy. We can employ a series of measures to alleviate the pain."

If you feel pain for more than a day or two, Dr. Torpey recommends creating a log of when the pain occurs so that the doctor can better understand what you are experiencing.

"When does this bother you?" he asks. "Is it during the day, at night, during an activity, when at rest, during chemo, immediately afterward? Is it aching or a sudden shot of pain? Does it happen out of the blue, or can you anticipate it based on other symptoms? Write it all down and bring the log to your doctors. We'll be in a better place to understand what is happening to you and can individualize treatment based on what you've observed."

Dr. Staats says pain intervention is broken into four general categories, starting with conservative treatments and moving gradually toward more aggressive or invasive procedures.

"Medication is the first response," he explains. "We employ everything from muscle relaxants and narcotic analgesics to anti-inflammatory analgesics to antidepressant or antiseizure medications. We can prescribe physical medicine strategies such as heat or ice, massage therapy, or electrical stimulation."

"There are two perspectives," Dr. Torpey says. "One is to focus on the pain, and the other is to focus on what we call comorbidities, which are other symptoms that are the result of the original pain."

Perhaps because your arm is aching, you've begun carrying groceries, laptops, or children only on one side. As a result, your back is beginning to give you problems.

"When pain is specific to a certain joint area, I generally initiate a course of physical therapy to maintain full motion of the joint and strength of the muscle group involved," says Dr. Torpey. "You want to reduce the swelling of any areas affected by the pain using ice, heat, or other modalities.

"You can also use pain patches such as Lidoderm," he says. "If you put that over the point where you ache, it can numb the area and give you a break from the pain."

"Moist heat helps soothe aches," says Dr. Weinrib. "When you're in spasm, the fibers of the muscle are very tight and short. As heat permeates the muscle, it releases the fibers, helps them open up, which increases the range of motion of every joint it's affecting."

Dr. Weinrib recommends buying an inexpensive clay pack called a hydrocolator, which is boiled, placed in towels, and then arranged over the area in pain.

"I suggest patients use it for ten to twenty minutes every two hours. If after removing it the area feels swelled, apply ice," she says. "The heat/ice approach improves circulation to the area, relieving pain and increasing flexibility."

Dr. Weinrib also recommends two homeopathic remedies, coconut oil or the analgesic aid Traumeel to augment your heat application.

"They're both wonderful for the skin and very gentle," she explains. "If you select Traumeel, apply it to the affected area before you put the hydrocolator on. If you use coconut oil, rub it into your skin after the treatment is over."

If after a few weeks of intervention the problem continues, Dr. Staats says psychological stress can amplify any biologic source of pain.

"The stress that comes as a result of cancer is very real and can create what are called negative states, which act like a magnifying glass on pain," he explains. "Most people have no idea that the area of the brain that processes depression is the same area that processes pain. So in 1996, I wrote a paper on the fact that pain may begin in your extremities, but in the end it really is all in your head."

For patients with depression and pain, Dr. Staats recommends antidepressant medications.

"Pain management today is an interdisciplinary practice," he says. "There's a fair amount of gestalt that goes along with diagnosis. If someone comes to me and they are clearly depressed about the pain they are in, I may be more likely to start them on an antidepressant because their symptoms will benefit from that medication more than an antiepileptic drug.

"Using this logic, a morbidly obese patient presenting pain would be better off with an antiseizure drug that will not cause weight gain," he continues.

If these remedies don't alleviate the muscle or bone discomfort, it may be time to get a little more aggressive about the situation.

"If medication and physical medicine strategies are not working, the next thing to try may be a neuroblockade," says Dr. Staats. "Sometimes if muscles go into spasm, we can inject a little bit of local anesthetic and a steroid into the muscle. This is a very common intervention method that many doctors use."

While the emphasis during pain management is to remain as noninvasive as possible, it may sometimes be necessary to deliver relief to the patient via devices or medications that are implanted inside the body.

"I'm a past president of a group that tries to improve pain through chemically or electrically modified nervous system intervention called the North American Neurological Invasive Society," says Dr. Staats.

Artificial devices can be placed in the spinal nervous system to charge the pathways of pain with a sensation of tingling or buzzing, which eliminates pain by creating feelings similar to a massage.

"The majority of pain receptors are in the spinal cord," Dr. Staats says. "There are literally hundreds of receptors, ion channels, transmitters, and reactions between different levels of the spinal cord that can be targeted with specific drugs.

"Before we implant, we put a catheter into the spinal fluid through a needle and allow the patient to test it for three or four days to see if it helps," says Dr. Staats. "While most chemo-induced pain will end when the treatment is over, there are some circumstances where nerve damage will continue to cause pain, and these types of procedures, while more extreme, can increase life expectancy and improve enjoyment considerably."

You don't have to suffer in pain. Keep that dialogue between your oncologist, your supporting medical team, and yourself open, and let them know when, where, and how something hurts. They will figure out what can be done to make you feel better.

Constipation/Diarrhea

If your particular chemotherapy regime commonly triggers constipation or diarrhea, your oncologist will let you know this before treatment begins. You'll receive recommendations for over-the-counter remedies along with prescription medications.

If you're constipated, help soften your stool by maintaining proper hydration. Include fiber in your diet. Exercise.

"By taking in adequate amounts of protein, fiber, and fluid, you'll withstand the side effects of cancer treatment much better than someone who doesn't pay attention to their diet," says nutritionist and dietitian Amy Bragagnini. "It's especially important to remain properly hydrated. Some side effects from chemotherapy make it challenging to consume enough fluid. Eight to twelve cups of liquid per day is recommended—water, 100 percent fruit juice, milk, or a sports drink are the suggested choices. Limit caffeinated beverages, soda, and alcohol. Try to find the liquid that works best for you."

If diarrhea is the problem, Amy suggests drinking plenty of fluids to replace those lost. In addition, she says, "Bananas, rice, applesauce, or white bread are all good choices. Avoid dairy products; greasy, fatty, spicy foods; or anything that contains alcohol or caffeine."

If you opt for a prescription or over-the-counter medication to deal with these symptoms, read the label carefully and follow directions exactly. Don't take anything unless your doctor has approved it.

Regardless of whether or not you are straining to have a bowel movement or find you cannot be far from a toilet, these side effects can be managed quite effectively if their presence is known. They can lead to complications if they are ignored. Do not suffer in silence. Speak up, and let the professionals lead you to relief.

Drowsiness/Insomnia

Sometimes during chemo it's hard to get through the day with your eyes fully open. Other times, you may find sleep to be as elusive as a leprechaun. Though these can each present their own separate challenges for a woman trying to keep her life as normal as possible, there are some simple solutions you can employ.

"You must respect your rhythm," says Dr. Canzone. "People forget that during treatment things can't really be the same as when they're not in treatment. I hear many patients saying that if they lie down in the middle of the day, it'll show that they're weak. And my response is that's okay. You are."

Dr. Canzone says the essential point in dealing with the side effects of your treatment is to listen to your body and provide what it is asking.

"Don't be afraid of it," she says. "Don't fight against it. Just try to let things flow."

It's probably your medications and your body's response

to them that is making you tired, but it could be stress or even depression. Fight back by staying active.

"You must motivate yourself," says Dr. Weinrib. "It's not about jogging a mile or doing something hard. You want to keep your circulation going so that you remain flexible.

"It's important to keep your mind alert too," she adds. "Do a crossword puzzle or talk with friends—anything that engages your brain and makes you think. Drinking green tea will help you stay alert, and physical activity will help you later on so that when bedtime arrives you're tired enough to sleep."

If you find yourself lying in bed and staring at the ceiling while the rest of the world falls off to sleep, there are ways beyond medication to help you relax.

"One of the things you can do is look at your bedroom," Dr. Weinrib suggests. "Is your bed comfortable or would it be better if you placed an egg crate, which is a soft foam pad, underneath the sheets? You may want to use pillows under your knees or between your knees, or perhaps have a cervical pillow underneath your neck to alleviate discomfort and make sleep easier to achieve."

"If you're having trouble sleeping, put lavender on the pillowcase," Dr. Wright suggests. "A lot of people find it to be very effective. I like that it's inexpensive and has no side effects."

"You want to prepare your body so that it is ready for sleep," says Dr. Canzone. "The basic concept here is winding down as the day goes along, and calming your system. Nighttime is not the time to be sitting at your computer or listening to jarring music. You need to relax. Move your mental state from alert and engaged to calmness and tranquility."

"When you head to your room at night, ask yourself if you're ready to sleep," Dr. Weinrib says. "Don't stick with old habits if they don't work right now. You may have always gone to bed at ten, but during chemo you may find you're not tired at that time. So do something else that's peaceful. Listen to music, or try a relaxation technique."

Dr. Canzone suggests that simple everyday herbs may help you work toward a night of rest. "You can use a pinch of nutmeg in a cup of hot milk, because nutmeg has sleeping properties in it. Poppy seeds are also helpful. Steep one teaspoon of poppy seeds in a cup of hot water for about six minutes, strain, add a teaspoon of honey and enjoy."

She also suggests that for those who find themselves unable to sleep, begin the winding down process in late afternoon.

"Have a cup of hot milk with nutmeg and honey at about five o'clock," she recommends. "Then have another cup right before bed. This will begin the calming process. You won't fall asleep after the first cup, but you'll start to feel the relaxation, and the winding down will continue into the evening."

If you're in bed and sleep still will not come, try Dr. Weinrib's visualization technique.

"Lie on your back in a very comfortable position," she says. "Breathe very slowly into your body, and then slowly bring that breath down to your feet, allowing yourself to feel the tension there. Exhale, and with that breath, release the tension in your feet. On the next inhale, breathe into your calves, your knees, your thighs, your pelvis. Work your way up the body with every intake of breath. Visualize the tension flowing away from you with every exhale.

"This is very effective," she says. "I would say half of my patients don't make it to the top of their head. They fall asleep and remain that way all night."

Former NFL star John Nies offers a variation on this approach. "Take very deep breaths," he says. "With each inhale, visualize a white healing light whose job is to cleanse the body of all cancer cells, negative thoughts, and feelings. Envision the white light permeating the entire body, making its way to the infected cells, collecting the intruders, and expelling them with each exhale.

"I recommend doing this for ten minutes," he says. "It's very soothing and healing and should help create a relaxed, tranquil state."

Sleeping pills are another option. If your doctor has recommended them to you, you can use them to get the sleep you need. Our experts agree, however, that the more naturally you fall asleep, the deeper and more complete your slumber will be.

"Sleep is essential to your overall health," Dr. Weinrib says. "As you sleep, things heal so much better. Your recovery time is better. There are several studies that show you lose wrinkles if you sleep more."

After a nighttime of rest, you'll not only feel better but odds are you'll look better too!

If you need a nap during the day, take one. It's not in your best interest to lie around all day every day, however.

Inertia won't maintain your flexibility, your strength, or your attitude.

When night approaches, be aware of your surroundings. As mentioned earlier, don't amp up your heart rate with violent television programs, pounding music, glaring computer screens, or challenging conversations. Imagine your body as a music box. As darkness falls, let the melody of your physical energy begin to slow down. By the time you are ready to close your eyes, the sounds of your day will be silenced and the symphony of sleep can rule.

Fatigue

Fatigue becomes more pronounced as chemotherapy continues and the cumulative effects of the medications begin to sap your energy. Maintaining the appropriate level of stamina to get you through your day becomes difficult. It may seem counterintuitive to push your tired body into activity, but this is the first and best step to overcoming weariness.

"Exercise will make you feel energized," John says. "A sedentary lifestyle will stagnate the body's energy, compromising your ability to heal."

"No matter how you're feeling when you begin," he continues, "if you make the effort to exert yourself, your mood will elevate. Your endorphins will flow. You will feel better, happier, and more in control of your body."

As a former professional athlete who now works with women facing disease, John says the benefits of daily activity are essential for those looking to improve their life situation.

"It doesn't matter if it's strenuous or moderate exertion or just walking," he says. "The sheer impact of being physically active has been proven to create strength, confidence, and energy no matter what the body is facing."

Dr. Wright agrees. "We offer a fitness program at our center because it's vitally important for patients to move and stretch and be as active as they can," he says. "Yoga is wonderful, as is Tai Chi. When people ask me what is best, I always quote Mark Twain—the surest way to kill yourself is live someone else's life. You can't let others decide what you need. You have to take all the advice out there, internalize it, and do what works for you."

If you've got dogs, get out and walk them. If there's a child in your life, put the child in a carriage and take a few turns around the neighborhood. Call a friend and go for an early morning stroll, or if the mood to get outside suddenly hits you, go for a walk by yourself. You can pick up yoga or low-impact aerobic tapes and DVDs at the library. You can garden or swim, rollerblade, ice skate, or take a bike ride. The goal is simply to get on your feet and move.

If you do, but still find you're fatigued, it's possible you're overdoing it or suffering perhaps from an underlying problem, such as depression, anemia, or pressure from a tumor.

"You need to know the cause of the fatigue," Dr. Weinrib says. "If you're eating a normal diet, doing normal exercise to keep your circulation up, and getting the right amount of sleep, then something else is working against you. It's important to know what that something is."

Dr. Weinrib recommends undergoing tests to eliminate the possibility of contributing medical conditions.

"If no medical intervention is required, I suggest starting an energy journal," she says. "Look at the times when your energy drops. Try to correlate that to the activities you're doing. You may find that you're doing things when your energy is low. If you work around your body's natural rhythm, you'll discover when you have more energy and can do more activities then."

If you find you have more pep early in the day, do more then. Leave the afternoons for rest and relaxation.

"Don't be such a creature of habit that you work against yourself," Dr. Weinrib advises. "You may have always done a lunchtime jog, but may have to move that to mornings if that's when your stamina is best."

Conduct a self-study, identify when you're feeling most vigorous, and use that time to fight back against fatigue. And when you're tired, rest. It's that simple. And it really is okay.

Headaches

A variety of reasons exist as to why you may experience headaches during chemo—dehydration, stress, nausea, or effects that are generally unpleasant following a dose of anticancer drugs.

If you're experiencing headaches, especially severe ones, tell your oncologist so that he or she can eliminate contributing factors that are more serious from the list of causes and prescribe appropriate medications.

Once your doctor has concluded there is not an additional health problem to treat, you can work on finding the relief that suits you best.

"You can do some self-massage," suggests Dr. Weinrib.

"Your scalp is a muscle, and a lot of tension resides there. Use a moist towel around your head, or an ice pack if it's a hot headache, and massage the fibers in your neck by moving your fingertips in a circular motion and applying gentle pressure.

"Start at the top of the neck, and use two fingers to move out toward the ears," she continues. "You can also rub Traumeel into the skin for some analgesic relief."

Neurologist and professor Dr. Noah Gilson says headaches during chemo are often the result of dehydration due to nausea.

"Staying hydrated makes a big difference," he says. "I recommend proper fluid intake as a first defense, especially if there's been pronounced bouts of nausea. If the patient cannot accept water or water is not helping the situation, drink electrolyte liquids such as Gatorade to regain proper levels of hydration."

Dr. Canzone says it may be poor nutrition that's causing the trouble.

"It could be what we call a blood deficiency headache," she explains. "There's not enough oxygen in the body. Foods like dates, berries, cherries, mangoes, seaweed, pomegranates, and bone marrow soups help to enrich your blood.

"Or you could have dry brain," she continues. "Massage the head with brahmi oil or coconut oil, or put a few drops of coconut oil or almond oil on a Q-tip. Tilt your head back, place the Q-tip inside each nostril, and gently sniff it up toward your brain. These simple solutions offer big help to both hot and cold headaches."

If you have a headache, and your oncologist-approved

intake of analgesics such as aspirin, ibuprofen, or aceta-
minophen is not providing the help you seek, your doctor
could write you a prescription for a Transcutaneous Elec-
tric Nerve Stimulator (TENS).

"It's a little use-at-home machine with stimulation pads
that deliver a mild current through the skin that interrupts
the pain signal and stimulates endorphin production," Dr.
Weinrib explains.

Before you purchase a TENS, check with your insurance
to see if it's a covered expense. Once you have your machine, your doctor will send you to a physical therapist for
training on where to place the stimulation pads.

Numbness/Neuropathy

In its zeal to kill off cancer cells, chemo can damage the
nerves that connect our central nervous system to our muscles, skin, and internal organs. When these nerve ends are
affected, tingling or numbness can occur. This is called peripheral neuropathy. It causes patients to feel desensitized
in their hands or feet or both, which are not able to relay
a sense of heat or cold to the brain accurately.

This condition can be serious. Doctors will often change
medications or reduce the dosage at the first sign of neuropathy.

"Chemo can interfere with the structures of the nerve
fibers," Dr. Gilson explains. "Patients may notice an altered
feeling in their extremities, a clumsiness in their ability to
use their hands or feet, or an overall uncomfortable sensation.

"The good news," he adds, is that "in most cases, patients fully recover once the contributing causes are eliminated.

"Control your sugar intake," Dr. Gilson advises. "Cut back on alcohol consumption. Most importantly, find out what if any underlying causes exist and get those conditions under control."

"Neuropathy can be multifactorial," Dr. Torpey says. "It may be the result of an underlying ailment that wasn't critically significant until chemo caused the problem to surface. The first order of business is a medical workup to make sure there are no underlying problems such as diabetes or improper nutrition."

A trip to a neurologist for diagnostic tests will discern if this neuropathy is caused by the chemo or if it's a long-standing issue from an underlying condition, such as diabetes.

"A patient undergoing chemo with a history of a 'bad neck' may in fact be a borderline diabetic with a disc irritation," Dr. Torpey explains. "The chemotherapy may have caused these factors to become more clinically symptomatic. By treating the diabetes, we can effectively address the neuropathy."

There are other ways to treat the condition, and special concerns to be aware of.

"I counsel people who have neuropathy to inspect the affected areas carefully every day to make sure they do not have any minor cuts or abrasions or blisters that can't be felt because of the desensitization," says Dr. Torpey. "This is especially important with chemo patients because they're immune compromised and are at risk for infection. There should be no compromises to the skin, no cracks between the toes. The only way to be sure of this is to check every day.

"Once neuropathy is confirmed," Dr. Torpey continues, "an occupational therapist can begin desensitization techniques, such as massage, hot soaks, and soft tissue stimulation to work through these hypersensitivities. Are the neuropathy symptoms chronic? Are they worse in the cold? If cold is a contributing factor, and you like the heat low in your home, a simple strategy could be raising the thermostat a bit."

Dr. Torpey maintains that proper nutritional habits and some prescription medications can offset peripheral nerve damage.

"Vitamin B6 and B12 are important," he says. "Your doctor may give you some medicines to diminish nerve inflammation. Some, such as certain epilepsy medications, work quite well to calm the nerve inflammation that usually affects the toes and fingers of neuropathy patients."

Some anti-inflammatory or antiseizure drugs can affect mood. Review the side effects with your doctor before deciding to take the medication, and pay attention to how you feel once you have begun. Keep your oncology team abreast of how you are coping with the side effects of the remedy, as well as the neuropathy itself.

Another approach, says renowned massage therapist, author, and teacher Gayle MacDonald, is to employ gentle massage. Reflexology (massage of the hands and feet) and Reiki (a Japanese form of healing intended to harmonize body, mind, and spirit through the hands of a trained practitioner) can provide temporary relief that, as Gayle says, "not only makes the patient feel better, it gives them hope by reminding them of what their body feels like to be normal."

Nausea

At least six out of every ten people receiving chemotherapy are expected to experience nausea and vomiting during their treatment. While that's a large percentage of patients, there are also a significant number of ways to cope with the situation.

A line of drugs known as antiemetics have proven so effective, many doctors now look at this once debilitating side effect as something they can do a lot to prevent. At the beginning of every infusion, you'll probably receive a series of preventative medications in your drip that will either drastically reduce the amount of time you spend sick or completely eliminate it all together.

No matter how scrupulously your oncologist works to protect you from the stress, anxiety, and exhaustion nausea produces, be prepared to face at least some vomiting and rocky stomach issues over the course of your chemo experience.

"Some drugs are more likely to cause nausea," says Dr. Canzone. "Your doctor will let you know if you are going to receive medications that do."

If your chemotherapy is on the top ten list of nausea producers, try drinking ginger tea.

"It works for many people," Dr. Wright says. "But if ginger is not a flavor you like, try Sea-Bands—another very effective way to control nausea."

Worn on the wrist, Sea-Bands use acupressure to block the transmission of nausea signals to the brain, thereby controlling the urge to vomit. They are completely natural, have zero side effects, and can be worn by anyone regardless of age, strength, or medical condition.

While statistically proven effective, Sea-Bands do not work for everyone. That is true of many of the remedies associated with cancer side effects—what works like a charm on one patient is completely ineffective on another. We have to do our part to seek out what is available and then try the remedies ourselves.

If you're throwing up while wearing Sea-Bands or find ginger tea undrinkable, there are more basic ways to control a sick stomach.

"The best treatment for nausea—and fatigue—is exercise," Dr. Wright says. "I give patients a pedometer and tell them to give me between five- and ten-thousand steps a day. If they do that, they're keeping up their end of the bargain. Their body will stay healthy."

Making sure you have a stomach full of the right kinds of foods will also make a huge difference in how well you tolerate infusions, both during treatment and in the days that follow.

"You have to understand why nausea happens," Dr. Canzone says. "You go for your chemo, and you're nervous. Perhaps you haven't eaten, or eaten very little, or eaten foods that are difficult to digest. You begin your infusion, and your body receives these incredibly powerful drugs either on an empty stomach or on top of foods that it cannot digest. Your body can't handle the stress. So what happens? You throw up."

Food choices are an easy, central way for all of us to take back some of the control cancer seems to hijack. If we're careful about what we put into our stomachs, we'll reap the rewards when our bodies have the resilience to accept the drugs we're pouring inside of us.

"Eat foods that are going to digest easily and gently nourish you," Dr. Canzone says. "It's a natural physical mechanism for your body to want to expel the drugs coming into you. Even though they're wonderful and are going to destroy your cancer, they're also highly toxic. So you have to make food choices that make sense."

Body Beautiful

Though you are dealing with the physical blow of cancer, everything you do to maintain your health during treatment will enhance your inner strength—and your physical beauty. Let go of the notion that it's selfish to put yourself first. Accept that during chemo, you must be your number-one priority. Allocate the time you need to take care of yourself, and let those who want to help you pick up the slack. You'll be doing everyone in your life a huge service by including them in your quest to be well.

If maintaining normalcy in your looks and life is one of your treatment goals, pay attention to what your body is telling you. Nourish it properly, speak up when something needs to be said, rely on your medical team to get you through chemo and its side effects, and concentrate your energy on the business of you.

If you allow yourself every opportunity to feel as well as you possibly can, your skin, your spirit, and your psyche will project the lovely radiance of calm, well-being, and contentment. What could be more beautiful?

To learn more about the information discussed in this chapter, please visit these websites:

www.cancer.org

csn.cancer.org

www.gildasclub.org

www.neuropathy.org

www.wegeinstitute.org

www.spineuniverse.com

www.bodycentralnyc.com

www.medicinehands.com

www.cherylchapman.com

www.njpowercenter.com

www.mayoclinic.com

CHAPTER 6

A Girl Thing

THE SURVIVORS REMEMBER

Marybeth: My treatment triggered menopause, and that, combined with steroids and poor food choices, piled twenty pounds on me. I'd always been athletic and fit, so this was hard for me to deal with. I worked out whenever I could, but it wasn't until chemo ended and I went on Weight Watchers that I was able to regain some control over my weight.

Chris: I gained forty pounds. Some of it was chemo, and some of it was my complete lack of exercise other than lifting my fork at the dinner table. I dieted after treatment, and lost twenty-five, which is fine. My skin cleared up too. Even though this was hard to deal with, it was all temporary.

Laura: It was important for me to be in control throughout my cancer. Staying in shape was the only way I could actually retain some control over my body, but I still lost about thirty-three pounds during treatment.

Patricia: My bones ached and the hot flashes from menopause were very frequent, but I took that as a good sign.
It meant my body didn't have any estrogen. I gained weight
and have had to work hard to get rid of the extra pounds,
but I think that would've happened to me anyway—my
body just slowed down faster because treatment put me
into early menopause.

The Side Effects

hot flashes	vaginal dryness
loss of appetite	yeast infections
mouth sores	bladder infections
reduced libido	compromised sexuality
weight gain	changes to taste
weight loss	

The Pearls

Chemo dishes out its rough blend of side effects on an
equal basis. Men get prostate and testicular cancer, women
get breast and ovarian. We each get as bald as the other.
Treatment isn't any kinder to male skin than it is to ours.

Our complex reproductive systems, however, provide many
more organs for cancer to affect. Feeding on hormones,
these cancers thrive on the biological fuel that powers our
female engines. The first thing chemotherapy does is starve
cancer of the food it needs to live by shutting down our
hormone producing capabilities. This is an incredible, life-

saving medical breakthrough. It's also why we suffer in unique ways our brothers in arms will never experience.

Enduring the sexual side effects of chemo can have a direct impact on how we look and feel. Aching bones and hot flashes have an impact on our posture, wardrobe, and attitude. Solving these problems restores our comfort and confidence. We feel better, we look better, and we radiate once again from within the feminine beauty that is our special domain.

WHAT'S GOING ON

Eliminating estrogen from our bodies is one of the most effective weapons oncologists use to halt a hormone-positive tumor in its tracks. Without this nourishment, the cancer cannot continue to exist. Highly effective chemo drugs wipe out malignant cells present in our bodies. Our empty hormone reserves make sure new tumor cells never get the opportunity to grow.

Our ovaries and vaginas depend on a regular supply of estrogen to operate properly. Without it, they shut down. Menstrual periods become irregular or completely disappear. The flesh inside our vaginas becomes thin and dry. Opportunistic infections arise. Struggling to replace the missing hormone, our pituitary gland sends an emergency signal to our ovaries to get to work. They do not respond. Moving into overdrive to conquer this breakdown, the heart races and the skin sweats, and we are left feeling clammy and cold. Emotions go haywire. Metabolism slows. We put on weight. We are not happy campers anymore.

These issues, though difficult for any woman to deal

with, hit chemo girls particularly hard. We're already doing all we can to fight the good fight. The last thing we want is a new combat front. These symptoms are also difficult for many women to discuss. Deeply private and personal, an intimate conversation with your oncologist about the state of your vagina, sexuality, bones, or periods might be hard for you to initiate.

"It's sometimes very embarrassing for a woman to discuss these issues with her oncologist, especially if he's a man," Dr. Thomas Caputo says. As chief of Gynecological Oncology at New York Hospital, Dr. Caputo treats hundreds of chemo girls annually. He's well acquainted with just about every sexual side effect they'll face. His overriding advice to these women is to understand that doctors are unfazed by these issues. They have much help to offer—if they know it's needed.

"Though it may be uncomfortable for you to talk about sexual issues or matters concerning your libido or vagina, if you are upfront with your caregivers, they should be able to help you overcome or at least cope with whatever it is that you are experiencing," says Dr. Caputo.

Modesty, dignity, shyness, and pride all have their place in our lives, but when it comes to the side effects of chemotherapy, it is almost impossible to imagine anyone on your oncology team being surprised by any symptom you report. It may be difficult to get the words out, but if you find the courage just to state your problem, you'll likely come away from the conversation with a solution or two that will help make a difference in how you feel, how you look, and how you carry on.

Hot Flashes

Shutting down hormone production usually throws a woman into menopause, which is the cessation of the menstrual period. Younger chemo girls (under 40) will likely resume their periods once treatment ends. The older the patient is, however, the greater her chance that chemo-induced menopause will remain permanent.

During treatment, it doesn't really matter whether your menopausal state will continue or end. Understanding and dealing with the symptoms is what's important.

The most well-known side effect of menopause is a hot flash. Your heart pounds, your body heats up, you sweat, your face turns red. As the flash subsides, a feeling of chilliness or clamminess occurs.

While there really isn't any way to stop a hot flash from happening, there are things you can do to make them less severe.

"Look for body-building foods," suggests Dr. Canzone, an Eastern medical doctor. "Try anti-inflammatory foods, such as asparagus, cabbage, brussels sprouts, cauliflower, broccoli, berries, dates, figs, avocado, fish, different summer squash, winter squash, green beans, root vegetables, whole grains, and lamb, because they will help your system adjust.

"Avoid vinegar, smoked foods, cashews, peanuts, and pistachios," she continues. "They cause inflammation, and what you want at this time are the more cooling foods in your system. Don't over acidify your body with heavy foods, fatty meats. If you don't digest and break down your foods, that can cause too much heat in your body and hot flashes."

Dietician and nutritionist Amy Bragagnini agrees that dietary changes may help. "Avoid hot spicy foods, alcohol, caffeine, hot beverages, and soups," she says. "Keep yourself hydrated. Soy contains estrogen-like compounds called isoflavones. It has been suggested that soy may help reduce hot flashes, but I would advise caution if you have had breast cancer. Ask your doctor if this is a safe choice for you.

"Your thyroid might be out of balance," Dr. Canzone adds. "Ask your doctor to run a full thyroid panel to make sure that's not the source of the problem."

"Reflexology and shiatsu are helpful because there's too much fire in the body, and it needs to be cooled," says massage therapist Gayle MacDonald.

Cheryl Chapman, a massage therapist specializing in oncology and mastectomy patients, agrees that massage helps. She advises using common sense and caution during the session.

"Warm oil will only make it worse," she says about massage practices. "Use cold stones on the face, in the hands. Let the massage lower the heart rate."

Infections

Without hormones producing the lubricating juices that keep our vagina and urinary tract in balance, bladder and yeast infections become more common. They are almost instantly recognizable. If you notice a discharge in your panties or feel a certain pressure in your abdomen, call the doctor. Quick intervention is the best way to stop these problems in their tracks. Once treated, there are several ways you can lessen your chances of getting another.

"Yeast infections are very common for some women, while others almost never get one. It's dependent on the chemistry of each woman's body," Dr. Caputo says. "To combat an occurrence, you can try taking acidophilus. Add yogurt and cranberry juice to your diet. Wear cotton underwear. Stay away from tight pants—give that area of your body a chance to breathe in clothes. Avoid harsh laundry detergents."

If you follow this advice and still end up with an infection, Dr. Caputo recommends prescription creams, oral medications, and nonsensitizing creams that can be applied to your vulva.

"Tell your doctor, or call your gynecologist—they can prescribe Diflucan or a symptom-appropriate medication," he says.

With bladder infections, Dr. Caputo says regular urination and lots of liquids are the best defense. "Go to the bathroom often. Don't hold it in. Urinate after sexual intercourse. If these infections become frequent, go to a urologist, who can examine you with a scope to ensure that there's not some contributing problem causing this to happen.

"Notify your oncologist the moment you feel an infection coming on," he adds. "Get on an antibiotic right away. That will knock the infection out."

Bone Density/Osteoporosis

Chemo drugs and estrogen-blocking hormone treatments are particularly effective in treating certain types of female-specific cancers. They also raise the likelihood of decreasing the mineral density in our bones, which leads to osteoporosis.

"Think of your bones as a bank for calcium," says orthopedic surgeon Dr. Brian Torpey. "The deposits you've made in terms of calcium intake throughout your life, as well as your level of physical activity, will determine your bone stock, as it's called. Chemo can be likened to a withdrawal from your stock—it reduces your calcium resources."

To replenish what chemotherapy is taking from your bones, Dr. Torpey advises eating the right foods and taking supplements.

"Maintain your intake of supplemental calcium around 1,000 to 1,500 milligrams per day. Supplemental vitamin D intake should include 200 to 800 IUs. Eat low-fat dairy products like cheese, milk, and yogurt. Include fresh fish, spinach, broccoli, and orange juice in your diet.

"Depending on your age, I would also recommend getting a baseline bone density reading before you begin your treatment so that the amount of calcium in the bones can be monitored," he adds. "Because of the long-term effects the patient may have to deal with once the cancer is gone, we like to make sure their bone strength is at appropriate levels. We want them to enjoy the rest of their lives without being frail or compromised."

Dr. Torpey says that the closer you are to menopause, the more important it is to get this baseline scan. If you're in your forties or fifties, ask your doctor about scheduling a scan. If you're in your thirties or younger, discuss risk factors including weight, ethnicity, and family background with your oncologist to decide when to schedule your base-line scan.

Sex

You may think that dealing with cancer means that your sex life is gone, but that's only true if you want it to be.

"If a woman is going through chemo, I recommend she send her partner for a massage," says Cheryl. "Everyone needs touch. They need contact. Massage is a good way to satisfy that skin hunger without any related intimacy."

"Real life is not like a Hollywood movie," Dr. Caputo says. "No one is having as much sex as we think they are. But intimacy is important. During cancer, it's not impossible to maintain a sexual relationship with your partner, as long as you don't pressure yourself into a state where you cannot function as a sexual being."

As a gynecological oncologist, Dr. Caputo is well versed in the various symptoms that could put the kibosh on physical intimacy during chemo.

"There is limited or no vaginal estrogen. The vagina becomes dry, making sex painful. Women may lose their interest in sex because it's uncomfortable, or they feel unattractive, or they're tired or stressed, or their hormones have been wiped out," he explains. "There are things we can do to help them, as long as they let us know this has become a problem.

"The first thing I tell all my patients is don't quit your job," Dr. Caputo says. "Try to keep your life as close to normal as you can. Exercise. Go out. Talk on the phone. Don't withdraw from the world. This will all affect how you feel about your life and yourself. Being isolated and unhappy is not conducive to propping up your libido."

You don't have to make love during treatment in order to be healthy. But if you find the stress of your illness and its effects on your love life are starting to affect your mate as well as your own heart, consider ways to rekindle intimacy.

Confronted with vaginal dryness, Dr. Canzone suggests vitamin E or coconut oil as an aid. "You can just insert it into your vagina with your fingers," she says. "Or let your partner. It's very light and it will help you feel more lubricated and comfortable."

Dr. Caputo agrees that creams and oils can be very helpful. "Use over-the-counter vaginal moisturizer or lubricant inserts. They provide appropriate levels of lubrication. They're nonhormonally active and nonirritating. Look for Replens or other products specifically designed to help vaginal tissue regain elasticity and moisture.

"Vaginal dilators help stretch the walls of the vagina," he says. "These can make intercourse more comfortable. You can use a lubricant that is not hormonally active."

Check with your doctor to see if these remedies are appropriate for you. You can also try yoga, meditation, and exercise as ways to bring your body back into a more normal state. This can help you maintain your relationship as a joyful, intimate partnership.

Eating Right/Staying Fit

The food choices you make during chemo will have a huge impact on your ability to deal with almost every aspect of your cancer experience.

"Nutrition is a huge part of cancer treatment," says Amy. "Proper nutrition can help people build strength, withstand the effects of cancer and treatment, and manage fatigue or prevent it from happening. Eat small meals. Get adequate protein, fiber, fluid, and nutrition into the diet. You'll be healthier, more upbeat, and feel better."

If you are what you eat, be a hero and put into your body the protein and fiber and liquid and vitamins it needs to withstand the chemo assault. A proper diet of smart, tasty ingredients will manifest itself in a very positive physical way. You'll look better, you'll feel better, and you'll *be* better if you feed yourself the smart way. Here's how.

Be Prepared

Keeping the right kinds of food in your house will make it easier for you to remain nutritionally balanced during your treatment.

"Doing the shopping and stocking the pantry and the freezer so that you have your favorite foods around and can eat when you don't feel like eating is really the key to success," says Amy. "Cook in advance. Have friends and family prep meals and store them in your freezer or fridge. Have a variety of choices available. This will make eating much easier."

"Ask friends to make soups for you," Dr. Canzone says. "Go around your town and find the restaurant with the best, freshest soups. Buy a week's worth so you always have something tasty and nutritious to eat. Make sure you freeze the soups in one cup containers so the soups do not sit in your refrigerator and spoil."

"You want to have enough choices so that something will spark your interest," Amy says. "Keep plenty of fruits and vegetables in stock, canned, frozen, or raw. They are good for vitamin and mineral intake."

"Whole grain breads are filling, easy to digest, and fiber rich," says New York–based chiropractor and nutritionist Dr. Joann Weinrib. "Rice and potatoes are easy to make and eat. Try to stay close to fresh. Watch your salt intake. That can dehydrate you at a time when you want to maintain hydration."

"You want to maintain a positive attitude and think that some of the harder side effects, like nausea, constipation, or diarrhea won't happen," Amy says. "But you also want to be able to combat those symptoms if they occur. A good way to do that is to be prepared with appropriate foods."

Eating Before Infusion

Going for treatment can be a nerve-racking business, especially if you're dealing with a lot of postinfusion side effects. Don't let your fears and anxieties get the better of your ability to eat.

"Be in nutritional training as you prepare for chemo," says Dr. Canzone. "If you properly nourish your system before your infusion, it's likely that some of the more difficult side effects such as nausea and vomiting can be lessened or even eliminated."

Dr. Canzone says brothy soups are a good choice the day before treatment. "Start off in the morning with a hot soup that is filled with nutrients—a chicken soup, a vegetable soup, or a tasty bone marrow broth," she advises. "These are calming to your system, because you don't have to work hard on digestion. These foods help ease you into your infusion by soothing your body while you feed it."

"As the day goes along, supplement with finger foods like dates and figs and avocado. Prepare a cold smoothie, something that's pleasant smelling and tastes good."

Amy agrees that it's important to consume easily digestible foods before heading to treatment. "A low-fat meal with a little bit of complex carbohydrate and a little bit of protein is the best," she says. "It can be as simple as a couple of pieces of whole grain toast with some peanut butter, a bowl of high-fiber cereal with low-fat milk and some juice, or egg whites and a bagel."

Never go to your infusion hungry or on an empty stomach, Dr. Canzone advises. "The drugs will gnaw at your stomach and cause all sorts of uncomfortable side effects.

"The biggest problem I find is that people don't nourish themselves enough to get through chemo," she says. "The taste buds are off. Treatment knocks out the appetite. While it's understandable not to want to eat, patients have to find a way to feed their bodies so that they can withstand the drugs they're receiving and continue to thrive.

"Dates, figs, and raisins take the decay out of the body. They are high in nutritional value," Dr. Canzone says. "They're also sweet and easy to eat. Even if you're very nerved up about the chemo to come, make a point to put something in your stomach before you go for your treatment.

The PMG nurses agree. "Eat a small meal to maintain your strength and protect your stomach," they advise. "Bring water or juice and some crackers with you so that you can continue to feed yourself lightly throughout your infusion."

"Stay away from preservatives and chemicals," Dr. Weinrib says. "Keep your food as close to fresh as possible."

Eating After Infusion

Once your treatment is over, you'll go home. Once there, continue on the path of small, easy meals and finger foods. Maintain a diet mix of protein, complex carbohydrates, and liquid.

"If your doctor has told you that you're going to be feeling bad for a few days after treatment, eat a little bit more leading up to infusion day to compensate for the days that follow when you don't want to eat as much," Amy says. "Try not to let your system become completely empty. You'll likely be more nauseated on an empty stomach than you would be if you had something small to eat."

"Try soups with protein and fiber," Dr. Weinrib says, "such as chicken and rice or noodles or beef broth and potatoes. Or buy some protein powder and mix it up with some yogurt and fruit in a shake."

"Treat yourself like a baby," Dr. Canzone says. "Would you feed a baby a steak? Even though you need to build up your blood, you have to do it in a way that's gentle to your system. Beef broth is great. A cold fruit smoothie without milk will help if you're nauseated or suffering digestive fire. Avoid dairy, as that could exacerbate the problem. Go in the opposite direction of what your stomach is feeling—if it's hot, give it cold foods. If it feels settled, try warm, gentle broth. As your body settles, introduce some poached salmon or some steamed vegetables, whatever you can handle that's not too rich."

"If you get home and can't eat, find a fluid with nutrients so that you receive some protein, vitamins, and minerals—something like a clear, liquid protein drink," says Amy.

If nausea is a problem, avoid hot foods or those with a strong odor. Go for either cold drinks or meals that can be served at room temperature—salads, pasta, cereals, figs, or dates.

"Concentrate on high-protein foods—lean meats, low-fat dairy products, egg or egg whites, beans, hummus, peanut butter, nuts, trail mix. Anything you can think of that will lend itself to getting more protein into your diet is good," Amy says.

"Don't forget about hydration," says Dr. Weinrib. "Gatorade or Pedialite are great. Seltzer water is a nice alternative to regular water, if you find that it's too heavy in your system. There is also coconut water, which has a lot of potassium and is gentle to your system. You can find it at health food stores."

Dr. Weinrib also recommends drinking green tea. "It's everything it's cracked up to be," she says. "It helps absorb oxidants, improves your healing quotient, fills you up, and is very soothing."

Since hydration is so crucially important right now, any-thing that drains your body of fluid is going to work against you. Avoid alcohol and caffeine and keep a glass of appro-priate liquid nearby.

"You don't have to drink the whole thing down in one sitting," says Dr. Weinrib. "Just have it nearby. Whenever you look at it, take a sip. By the end of the day, you should have taken in about six to eight glasses."

To make sure you're properly hydrated, look at your urine. "It should be lightly colored," says Amy, "If it's a dark amber, you may not be getting enough fluid."

Dry mouth and cracked lips may signal a lack of ade-quate moisture. If you're experiencing this or your urine is very dark, ask your oncology team about your kidney lev-els. They are a good indicator of your body's hydration.

As you move away from infusion day, keep the food and liquid flowing into your system. This is the proven path to overcoming the hardest effects of chemo. It gives your body the tools it needs to recover.

Putting on the Pounds

Though you may have imagined that chemo would shrink you down a size or two, many women find they gain weight during treatment. There are a variety of reasons for this—fluid retention, steroids, menopause, lack of exercise, and poor food choices are some of the most obvious. If you want to keep your weight in check, safe and sensible ap-proaches are the best way to begin.

"Eliminate salt," says Dr. Weinrib. "Go through all your foods and make sure nothing has salt. Chips, pretzels, hot dogs are all loaded with sodium. You want your intake to be close to zero. Any one item that's over 400 milligrams is too much."

"If you're gaining weight, do a dietary recall to find out what, when, and why you're eating," says Amy. "Are your habits emotionally based? Are you eating out of boredom or stress? Are you skipping meals? Try eating lots of small meals throughout the day. Never skip breakfast. It kick-starts your metabolism. Even if it's just a little bit of yogurt, or a protein bar, or a few crackers with peanut butter, put something in your stomach in the morning. That sets the nutritional tone for the rest of the day."

Another commonsense approach to weight control is staying active.

"Daily physical activity can elevate your immune system and keeps lean body mass strong. It can help improve appetite and elevate mood," Amy says. "Speak with your doctor first about your exercise/activity plans."

"Even though we all have different strengths and weaknesses as well as different attitudes about exercise, it's absolutely essential for anyone who wants to restore their vitality to partake in some sort of daily physical activity," says former NFL star John Nies.

"You don't want to push yourself too hard," he continues. "Move, stretch, increase your heart rate, and exert some effort on behalf of your body. Don't think of it as a chore, but as a blessing that you are able to move, and breathe, and engage in physical activity. Think of your body as a precious jewel or a holy temple. Treat it with love and respect. It will respond in a positive way."

The Skinny on Weight Loss

Some chemo girls experience significant weight loss during their treatment. If this happens to you, make sure you minimize the depletion of lean body mass.

"High calorie, high protein, nutrient dense foods should be eaten," says Amy. "Eggs and dairy and lean meats are all good sources of protein. Make sure you're eating every two to three hours through the day. If you find you don't want to chew, utilize supplement drinks. Find recipes online for high-calorie smoothies that contain flax seed, milk, oatmeal, fruit—anything that you can put into a blender to pump up calories and taste will create a drink that's satisfying and nutritionally sound."

"I ask my patients to drink a milkshake if they aren't nauseated," Dr. Canzone says. "Sometimes they'll protest and say they contain sugar, but sugar is okay, as long as it's not overdone. It's better to drink a milkshake than to stare at a plate of food and not eat any of it.

"Feed yourself the things your body can handle," she continues. "Treat yourself kindly. Focus on what is still wonderful about you. This will help offset the feelings of nausea, fatigue, and malaise that often wreck an appetite. If you create calmness in your whole being, you'll find your desire for food returning. By eating gentle, nourishing meals, you'll go a long way toward maintaining your health and your physical and spiritual balance."

Changes to Taste

As chemo continues, you may find your taste buds responding to foods differently, or not responding at all. While this makes it harder to eat, there are some strategies you can employ to offset the problem and maintain a reasonably healthy diet.

"Try experimenting with different flavors, seasonings, dressings, and marinades," Amy says. "Anything that will give moisture to food can help improve flavor and assist with ease of swallowing."

Amy recommends citrus, such as lemon or lime squirted on meat, because these fruits have a flavor even the most challenged mouth will be able to taste.

"Good mouth care is also important," she adds. "Rinse your mouth with baking soda and water to keep your mouth moist, clean, and healthy."

If you are experiencing a metallic taste, avoid canned foods. Switch to plastic eating utensils.

"Sometimes a metal fork or spoon adds to the offensive sensation," Amy explains. "You want to stay away from anything that is aluminum or metal or silver. Go for a more taste-neutral plastic."

If you develop mouth sores, "Try sucking on an ice pop during infusion," the PMG nurses recommend. "They'll hydrate you and help eliminate sores."

Dr. Leonard Wright says tea tree oil will also help alleviate this symptom. "Dilute it with water and swish it around in your mouth. The sores or lesions will clear up quite nicely."

The Rainbow Connection

No matter what your diet was like before cancer, pay attention to what you're feeding your body during treatment.

These choices have a direct effect on your health during chemo and in the years that follow.

"Definitive research shows that the best way to ensure proper nutrition and physical well-being is to get more fruits and vegetables into our diets," Amy says. "Go for extra fruits and veggies. Make a rainbow plate, with dark green leaves or vegetables, carrots, yellow bell peppers, or multicolored fruit salads. Consume a variety of fruits and vegetables, whole grains, lean meats, nuts or seeds, and low-fat dairy every day."

"Take a good supplement that has the full spectrum of minerals and vitamins," Dr. Weinrib says. "Don't depend on them to provide you with appropriate nutrition. Use them to help build up your reserves. Get the majority of your nutrients from food, not vitamins."

Amy agrees. "If you want to maintain good health and good strength and withstand the effects of chemo, make sure you eat well." If you need information on how to do this, contact a registered dietitian at your treatment center.

She also recommends contacting these sources for further nutritional advice:

- The American Dietetic Association

- The American Cancer Society

- The American Institute for Cancer Research

- www.eatright.org

- www.cancernutrition.com

"That last one is an oncology dietitian website with lots of great information," Amy says.

Nutritional Beauty

Eating well is an obligation we must fulfill if we're to get through chemotherapy with strength and resilience. The food choices we make have an instant effect on our ability to heal and manage our situation. Being hungry or malnourished leaves us weak, anxious, tired, and confused. Proper nourishment elevates our mood, raises our coping skills, and enhances our sense of personal power. Chemo girls can greatly enhance their fabulousness by making a commitment to ingesting the protein, fiber, vitamins, and minerals our bodies crave. Friends, family, and others who want to help you can lend a hand in this area by dropping off meals you and those you live with can enjoy.

Reaching out to your circle of supporters will go a long way toward making sure you receive your daily bread, giving them the opportunity to do something truly important and useful for you.

Enhance your physical fitness, elevate your spirit, and brighten your inner glow. Serve yourself the gift of nutritional health, and you'll dish out a message of positive energy to everyone who cares about you. Your hydrated skin, sparkling eyes, and honest smile will prove you can do more than survive under the enormous pressure of cancer treatment. You can thrive.

If we are what we eat, eat smart. Eat well. Your body will thank you—and your deepest beauty will continue to shine through.

To learn more about the topics discussed in this chapter, please visit these websites:

www.cancer.org

csn.cancer.org

www.bodycentralnyc.com

www.medicinehands.com

www.cherylchapman.com

www.cancernutritioninfo.com

www.aicr.org

www.eatright.org

www.healthcastle.com

www.njpowercenter.com

www.naturedoc.org

www.massagesource.com

www.mayoclinic.com

www.wegeinstitute.org

CHAPTER 7

The Integrative Approach

The Pearls

Choices in cancer treatment have vastly increased over the years. Surgery has become less invasive. Chemotherapy treatments are not as harsh. The practice of integrative medicine has dramatically increased.

Once misunderstood or rejected by a majority of Western medical practitioners, this type of medicine—known as alternative, complimentary, holistic, Eastern, or Oriental—is now offered in many major cancer centers across the country. New programs are being developed and implemented in oncology practices both large and small. Doctors who once viewed such practices as unproven or unreliable are being trained in acupuncture, massage, and meditation techniques. Large percentages of these doctors report that offering these treatment options to their patients improves the care they offer, as well as their own professional satisfaction.

"The goal of employing Eastern medical practices is to

treat patients with procedures that work, have little or no side effects, and are far less expensive than regular drug therapies," Dr. Leonard Wright says. "We find many Eastern practices to be extremely effective. Overall, our patients prefer to be treated with these more holistic approaches whenever they have a choice."

WHAT'S GOING ON

Integrative medicine marries the best and most effective of holistic Eastern medical practices with the technology-driven practices of Western medicine. Adopting therapies such as acupuncture, massage, meditation, and nutritional guidance into chemotherapy regimes creates a harmonious blend of treatments. Patients have choices and options that offer relief without additional drugs, chemicals, or side effects.

"Eastern medicine offers a respectful way of helping someone go through the process of coming back to health after a cancer diagnosis," Dr. Canzone, who practices Eastern medicine, says.

That respect, she says, includes the patient's decision to receive chemotherapy to destroy their cancer.

"If a patient of mine is receiving chemo, I know my job is not to treat the cancer because that's already being treated," Dr. Canzone explains. "My job is to build up the person. Listen to what she needs. Help her with diet and food so she is properly nourished. Provide massage and acupuncture to keep her energy strong and help her nausea go down."

"It's not about taking a lot of herbal formulas," Dr. Canzone says. "It's about healing the person who is holding the cancer."

The Alternative Approach

"The intent of an integrative practice is exactly what it says—to integrate the best of established Western medicine with the time-tested practices of Eastern philosophies," Dr. Wright says. "The goals are simple—to treat any symptoms the patient is reporting with alternative therapies that have proven to be effective."

A 1993 study revealed that one in three Americans used alternative or complimentary therapies as part of their medical care. This landmark report opened the concept of treating the whole person with a combination of modern and ancient practices to millions of patients who had never before considered such treatments effective. Demand for these therapies increased. Major medical centers responded by adding Eastern practices to their treatment roster. Western doctors began learning the age-old practices. Since that 1993 study was released, the number of U.S. hospitals and medical facilities offering integrative medicine has doubled. The trend continues to grow.

"There is very little risk or potential harm for the patient," Dr. Wright says. "We encourage them to try different therapies. We find helping them explore and find an individual therapy that works for them to be very satisfying for both the patient and the medical team."

Once considered a fringe element in medicine, integrative practices are now part of the mainstream cancer treatment in many of the country's leading hospitals and treatment centers. Holistic remedies are offered alongside traditional Western therapies. While there is some debate as to how effective these solutions are, if you are experiencing side effects and are not happy taking additional drugs, ask your oncologist about integrative medicine. You may discover a whole new world of treatment options to help you in your quest to be well.

Acupuncture—A Point of Relief

"Acupuncture is a practice of assessing the patient in a non-Western, energetic way," Dr. Wright says. "Through careful history taking, the use of pulse and tongue diagnosis, and O-ring testing, a plan can be made and then needles placed in the appropriate meridians to change and redirect the body's energy. When the treatment is complete, the pulse is rechecked to assess the patient's response."

"It's my first choice for nausea intervention," he continues. "I can look any patient in the eye and tell her we have a very good chance of improving her condition, with little or no chance of hurting her or making her condition worse."

Based on the principal of universal life energy inside each person, acupuncture is an ancient Chinese practice that moves blocked or restricted energy in the body, known as chi or qi, so that normal functions are restored.

"There are twelve energy tracks in the body called meridians," Dr. Wright explains. "Think of chi as an underground system of energy. The meridians are points in the body, like Old Faithful in Yellowstone National Park, where the energy comes to the surface."

"Acupuncture is simply inserting a needle into these meridian points to redirect the body's energy," he continues. "With my knowledge of these points, I can assess the patient in a different way than Western medicine. By doing a pulse diagnosis and asking various questioners, I can discover where the energy variations are, address these deficits, and then recheck the pulse."

"It's like dialing into your body's phone number for the day and reminding it of what it's supposed to do," Dr. Canzone says. "It helps the body absorb nutrients. It relieves nausea and stress and depression. It calms and refreshes.

"You know how you feel after a nice walk in nature?" she asks. "That's what acupuncture gives you—a gentle hum."

Dr. Wright says acupuncture's effects are immediate, but the trick is seeing how long the energy continues on its redirected path.

"It's very gratifying that with just a few needles you can change someone's energy flow. The question is how long does the change stay in effect? Some people don't hold the change," he says. "Those people typically don't do well with acupuncture."

"One of the interesting things about acupuncture is that it works on the same spots Western medical doctors call trigger points," says pain specialist Dr. Peter Staats. "We don't understand why it works, but it can be very beneficial to some patients.

"It's completely safe," Dr. Staats continues. "My concern is that patients be realistic about the effects. If you find relief, keep at it. If after five sessions you're not any better off than you were before, you may not want to continue, especially if it's not covered by insurance. It becomes a financial drain that isn't paying off in better care."

Unlike hypodermic needles, which are sharp and hollow to deliver blood or medicines into muscles or veins, acupuncture needles are solid and designed to go through just a couple of layers of skin. There is no pain associated with their use.

"The biggest question you want answered is does the practitioner use disposable needles," says Dr. Wright. "The only way this can hurt you is if needles are reused."

Acupressure is another ancient Chinese practice. Your fingers stimulate the redirection of energy. Gentle, firm pressure is applied to key points on your skin.

"Sea Bands are a great example of acupressure in action," Dr. Wright says. "The small knob on the wrist band is placed over the meridian point that controls nausea. By applying pressure in that spot, many people find relief.

"I teach my patients how to access certain points so they can help themselves," he says. "It's very effective and empowering for them to be able to aid in the redirection of their body's life force. They learn to participate hands-on in their own healing."

The Human Touch

Think of rubbing your temples when a headache strikes, and you'll have the basic idea behind acupressure. Headaches are particularly susceptible to the healing effects of both acupuncture and acupressure. They can also be relieved with gentle massage therapy.

"Headaches are often caused by stress and tension," says

Cheryl Chapman, a massage therapist specializing in oncology and mastectomy patients. "If you relax the muscles and ease the tension in the head and the shoulders with a good massage, you'll experience a lot of relief."

"Massage reduces pain and anxiety," says massage therapist Gayle MacDonald. "It improves your energy levels and reduces nausea for some people. Most importantly, it provides an emotional connection between the person with cancer and others."

Gayle says that physical contact is crucial for people whose sense of self and self-worth may be challenged by cancer treatment.

"Many people undergoing cancer treatment feel untouchable," Gayle says. "They disconnect from their bodies. Massage is a way to remember that your body can still be a source of pleasure—a place you can be comfortable within. Skin-to-skin contact between human beings is very healing to the heart."

As the author of two books on medical massage and a leading oncology massage instructor in the United States, Gayle has a deep knowledge of the benefits of massage for oncology patients.

"Our bodies are not just a mass of bones and blood and body tissue," she says. "There is an emotional part, an intellectual part, and a spiritual part. Since emotions lodge in the tissue, massage is a brilliant and effective way to address all these different components of the whole person."

"Cancer is such a stressful experience," says Cheryl. "Patients need to seek out therapies that provide relaxation. Massage is a wonderful way to put you in a different space, to diminish the problems of nausea and fatigue. It can really act as an integral part of cancer-pain management."

Oncology massage is a specific field where licensed therapists are trained over the course of forty- to fifty-hour seminars in exactly how to touch a cancer patient so that she reaps the healing rewards of therapy without any harm being done to her lymphatic system.

"A typical massage is a fairly vigorous event," Gayle says. "But when you're going through chemo, the intent must be to soothe and nourish. At most, the massage should go no deeper than the superficial layer of muscles under the skin. It is here that contact will be made with the nervous system. Long, gliding strokes will create a space of calm and tranquility for the client."

Regular massage aims to send the body's toxins through the lymph system. Oncology massage aims to do just the opposite. It's detrimental to have a patient's lymphatic system stimulated through forceful manipulation of muscles and joints when they're already overdosing on chemo toxins.

"If massage is too heavy, too strong, it will make the chemo patient feel even more tired or flu-like. You don't need additional toxins stirred up in the body," Gayle warns.

"Your chemo is breaking down the tumor, and those by-products don't just disappear," she explains. "They have to be metabolized through the lymphatic system, which is already handling a significant toxin load from the chemotherapy. Don't add to that by trying to detoxify your body through deep massage."

"Chemo patients simply can't tolerate a standard massage because the drugs break down the body's systems," says Cheryl. "The body's fluids and toxins are moved around with regular massage and excreted through the liver. The liver is already on overload from the chemo. You end up with a backlog of toxins in your body with no way to release them.

"It's like rinsing your clothes in the dirty water you just washed them in," Cheryl says of vigorous massage during chemo. "You're not going to get what you're looking for. You're going to end up with something you don't want at all."

No one dealing with cancer wants to walk away from a therapy feeling worse than she did on arrival. Anyone considering massage therapy must find a practitioner who is trained in working with cancer patients, or patients who are medically frail.

"If they have training in oncology massage, they should know what to do," Dr. Canzone says. "Similarly, they might have had training in craniosacral therapy, Reiki, or therapeutic touch—these modalities, though not cancer specific, suggest that the practitioner understands the importance of applying gentle, soothing pressure. Their clients will leave the massage session feeling energized, positive, and hopeful, not beaten down."

The benefits of therapeutic oncology massage are significant and can be taken advantage of as soon as you learn your diagnosis.

"The whole purpose is nurturing, caring, reducing stress, listening," says Cheryl. "Once you hear you've got cancer, you start to stress. The tension builds up. By the time you're ready for chemo, you're already in a taut, nervous state.

"By beginning a weekly course of therapy right away,

even before you've had surgery or seen a lot of doctors, you get out in front of the cancer and start to work toward a deeper wellness," she says. "The massage room is a safe place where a woman can cry, or swear, or forget about her kids and her spouse. She can put all her troubles away. For that hour, someone is taking care of her."

"Once you receive a cancer diagnosis, there is so much fear," Gayle says. "The mind is racing, you're trying to figure out what to do, who to turn to. Massage can be so helpful. It calms you down, so you make better decisions. I think once a week is best, but even if you have a massage after infusion, say every three weeks, you'll feel physically, emotionally, and spiritually better. It will rebuild trust in your body to have someone handle it in a reverent way."

"The benefits are substantial," Dr. Canzone says. "The oils used can nourish the tissues and make them stronger. Mahanarayan oil is good for brittle bones, neuropathy, and pain in the bones. Get some sesame oil, coconut oil, brahmi oil, or almond oil, and you can do self-massage to address some of the specific problems you have."

"The scientific research is very clear about massage reducing pain and anxiety," Gayle notes.

"The goal is to lower your cortisol level, which is the stress hormone; to engage the parasympathetic nervous system, which is your relaxation response; and to lower your blood pressure and heart rate," explains Cheryl. "It elevates the endorphin levels. You come away refreshed and revived and ready to continue your journey to wellness with a song in your heart, not a screech."

The Sound of Music

Soothing sounds have been proven to have a healing effect on human cancer cells, leading to a relatively new way to help alleviate the negative state of mind this disease can produce: music therapy.

An easy, inexpensive approach to helping patients cope with the emotional and physical upheaval of their diagnosis and treatment, music therapy is catching on in major medical centers all over the country. Trained music therapists work directly with patients to help them get through challenging situations. Whether or not this therapy is part of your oncology team's practice, you can still reap the healing benefits of music right in your own home.

"Our life is built on vibration and on sound," Dr. Canzone says, "Research shows cancer cells imploding on each other when classical music or healing chants are performed.

"Think about what happens to you when you awaken each morning," she continues. "If you turn on the news and hear about a fatality, or a terrorist threat, or something negative about politics, you start your day in turmoil and negativity. If when you rise you play classical music, or a Buddhist chant, or healing ragas, those sounds will play inside your brain all day. They will bring calmness to your being. This is a goal of the spiritual practice in Eastern medicine."

"Get a chime with a beautiful sound that touches you," suggests Cheryl. "Whenever you begin to feel like you can't deal with what's happening, ring that chime. This will break the negativity of the moment and center you in the present.

"Find music that soothes you," she continues. "While you're listening to it, imagine you're in a favorite place. It can be the beach, or the mountains, or perhaps in the arms of someone you loved long ago. Let that visualization take you away from your fears and troubles. It won't last forever, but momentary events like these will help you get through the day."

"Music therapy is very helpful," Dr. Wright says. "There are some instruments that are perfect for this because they encompass the whole scale. Its use is appropriate for cancer patients, as it can help them with their body's rhythm. My advice is to seek out professionals who are accredited at what you want them to do. Know that in this area of care, as well as all others, you're in good hands."

Finding Integrative Caregivers

No matter what your choice of medicine is called—Eastern, Western, alternative, holistic, Oriental, or something else—be sure that the people you work with are accredited, licensed, certified, or recognized by your state as professionals capable and experienced in the therapy they offer.

To begin a search for integrated caregivers, Dr. Wright suggests looking up the nearest major medical centers or consulting with the Society for Integrative Oncology. Learn from them where you can find practitioners in your area.

For Western medical acupuncturists, he recommends checking first with your state to see if there is a licensing board. Many states are beginning to create licensing legis-

lation. California and New York already have such requirements in place. If your state issues acupuncture licenses,
begin your search by considering only those who hold that
certification.

You can also contact the Academy of Medical Acupuncturists, of which Dr. Wright is a diplomat. Ask them to recommend practitioners in your area.

"They have to have the appropriate training and years
of experience, and passed the board exam, which is quite
rigorous," Dr. Wright says. "All members are very qualified.
You can feel confident engaging them."

Dr. Wright says there is a similar certification process for
Eastern or Oriental providers through the National Certification Commission for Acupuncture Oriental Medicine
(NCCAOM). They have a standard for education, training,
and experience all members must meet.

Dr. Canzone seconds that advice and recommends working only with NCCOAM acupuncturists.

"When you interview potential caregivers, ask them if
they are willing to work with your oncology team," she says.
"Do they respect the process of treatment you have chosen? Are they willing to work within the parameters of Western medicine? If they say yes and you feel they would be
right for you, introduce them to your doctors. They should
feel comfortable speaking with your Western medical practitioners. There shouldn't be any tension among the members
of your team because you've chosen to include alternative
approaches in your care."

Dr. Canzone strongly advises chemo girls to tell their oncologists about their acupuncture plans. "Never lie to your

doctor or withhold information about your activities. Select caregivers who can be flexible enough to understand your needs and wishes and help you achieve them."

If you'd like to receive massage during treatment, Gayle advises careful screening of therapists. "You should be comfortable during the massage," she says. "If you are not, and the therapist is unable to make the adjustments you have requested, stop the session.

"The Society for Oncology Massage (*www.S4OM.org*) may have therapists from your area listed in their Locator Service," says Gayle.

Questions to Ask When Interviewing Massage Therapists

1. What types of massage or touch therapies have you been trained in?
2. What kind of training have you done to work with someone with a history of cancer?
3. What type of precautions would you take for me? (Describe your treatment to them and explain the side effects you are experiencing.)
4. What type of clients do you most often work with? (Ideally they are people who require special adjustments such as infants, the elderly, or those with serious illness.)

"Ask potential therapists if they have direct experience working with cancer patients," Dr. Canzone says. "Do they understand what a port or a shunt is? Do they know what lymphedema is? Do they know what it looks like when someone's scar tissue has become septic?"

"Someone who doesn't understand these questions should not massage you," Gayle warns. "During treatment for cancer, a massage that causes pain, discomfort, or fatigue is worse than no massage at all. You need a massage therapist who appreciates the special needs cancer patients have, such as fragile bones, compromised lymphatic system, or low platelet count."

Easing Dis-Ease

The benefits of integrative care may lighten your cancer journey, but success and relief will occur only if you select the right practitioners. Just as you took the time and energy to put together your oncology team, you must be willing to devote an equal amount of focus to selecting alternative therapy providers.

Much of this work can be accomplished via a phone and the Internet. Turn on your computer, search for these societies and practitioners, and start making calls. Discuss the advantages and disadvantages of such caregivers with your oncologist. Once you locate therapists who can aid you in your quest to be well, integrate their presence into your Western medical team. Confirm with your chemo doctor that these practices will not put your body at odds with the chemo drugs it is receiving. Above all, be upfront with your practitioner—and yourself—about how these therapies make you feel. Only you can know if acupuncture, acupressure, massage, or yoga is achieving its desired effect.

Integrative medicine is focused on tapping the strength we maintain within our bodies during illness to recapture the physical and emotional harmony upended by our diagnosis.

"The power of life itself is an amazing gift, and that joy in our existence is what we want to recapture," Dr. Canzone explains. "In Eastern medicine, we consider sickness in the body not as disease, but rather dis-ease. It's your body in chaos, with self-awareness lost. We try to engender a sense of joy and cultivate the connection back to self."

"The holistic nature of Oriental medicine was its major draw for me," Dr. Wright says. "When I was diagnosed with a brain tumor, I wanted to be treated as a whole person, not just a man with a malfunction in one of my organs. I found the idea of myself as a vessel holding energy that needed to be redirected more appealing than the traditional Western medical view suggesting I was a broken machine that needed to be fixed."

Dr. Wright says that the melding of Eastern and Western practices into an integrative whole is why he is alive and well, and practicing medicine today.

"Western diagnostic techniques are by far the greatest, most dependable, and accurate mechanisms for identifying diseases that exist," he says. "If a person is manifesting symptoms, Western medicine can pinpoint to a greater degree of accuracy what is causing these symptoms in the body.

"Once we know what is wrong and begin a course of treatment, I think any patient will benefit from incorporating alternative therapies into their care," he continues.

"These therapies focus on the whole being. They recognize that our minds and spirits are as much a part of ourselves as our blood and our organs."

When he became ill, Dr. Wright says he could not find a Western medical team to help him.

"I was forced to find an alternative way to treat myself so I would get better," he explains. "What I found is that there is so much out there that has the potential to work, but the key word there is potential.

"You owe it to yourself to work at your own recovery," Dr. Wright says. "Find doctors who are open minded enough to allow you to explore all the possibilities. If you're considering alternative therapies, keep things as inexpensive and free of side effects as you can. Then you can experiment until you find the methods that work for you."

"It is important to feel good about your treatment, about your choices, about who you are in this moment of life," says Dr. Canzone. "Think about what you do to cultivate joy in yourself. Is there a psalm that brings you peace? Is there a song or chant that calms you? When your mind starts to turn toward fear and negativity, you are turning away from peace. You are cultivating dis-ease."

"Seek out that which will bring calmness to your being," she advises. "Embrace your life, spirituality, and essential oneness with everything around you. You will find the expressions of joy and wonder everywhere."

You are a living being with value and importance that goes beyond physicality. Imagine every cell in your body as an impression of life. Envision your essence as one of health and vitality. Reject the notion of dis-ease and focus on your return to wellness.

Once you have centered your inner eye on the positive elements of your life, you'll be able to visualize your body whole, healthy, and cancer free. Believe in your personal power. Seek tranquility. Maintain peace in your heart. Your body will grow in strength and calm and beauty. One day, you'll look back on this time with a sense of wonder that you made it, gratitude for your triumph, and a profound sense of the possibilities yet to come.

To learn more about the information discussed in this chapter, please visit these websites:

www.cancer.org

csn.cancer.org

www.integrativeonc.org

www.medicalacupuncture.org

www.aaom.com

www.nccaom.org

www.srom.org

www.wegeinstitute.org

www.spineuniverse.com

www.bodycentralnyc.com

www.medicinehands.com

www.cherylchapman.com

www.naturedoc.org

www.massagesource.com

www.mayoclinic.com

CHAPTER 8

Keeping the Faith

THE SURVIVORS REMEMBER

Marybeth: Getting sick rocked the trust I had in my body. Coming to terms with my own fallibility—and mortality—was a process that took some time. I had to learn to forgive myself for getting cancer and let go of the guilt I felt for causing so much anguish to my loved ones. But once I managed to put my disease in perspective, I began to see cancer as a blessing. Through it, I learned how to relax about my life and find peace in my soul.

Chris: When it happened, I asked myself how I felt about dying. I could see myself slipping over a threshold, with things being very peaceful, and I was not afraid to go there. But I made up my mind that it wasn't my time. And I was right. It wasn't.

Laura: Cancer was one of the best experiences that I have been through. I met the most amazing physicians and the most incredible patients. I know what it takes to survive, and I know how important and how wonderful life is. I make the most of every moment and cherish the gifts I have been given. I also know how lucky I am.

Patricia: A friend gave me a CD of the Brooklyn Tabernacle Choir, and I found it very peaceful and soothing to listen to while driving to work. A patient gave me a Papal Blessing, which I framed and put on my night table, next to a statue of Padre Pio, a Roman Catholic saint who believed that suffering all things for the sake of God was the way for the soul to reach God and who founded a home to relieve suffering. Since one of the biggest challenges for me was the lack of control I had over my body and my life, one of my most important lessons was learning how to put my fear, and my trust, in God's hands.

Rosemarie: I was raised as a Roman Catholic, and when this first happened to me, I was very angry with God. It wasn't until my second bout that I began to consider spiritual issues in a different way. With the help of my husband, who practices Zen Buddhism, I found a way to meld my traditional faith with a more Zen-like approach to prayer and spirituality. I'm still a Catholic, but I have a deeper way of looking at things now that goes beyond categories.

The Pearls

Learning that there is a cancer inside our bodies is one of the most devastating, life-altering events we will ever experience. Receiving this diagnosis is like having an explosion go off in our heads—we can't seem to hear beyond the roar of emotions washing over our brains—a furor of confusion and disbelief. Waves of resentment and anger may flood our minds. We may find ourselves drowning in a swamp of guilt or sinking under a tide of debilitating fear.

But as crazy as this may initially sound, some patients view—or over the course of their treatment learn to experience—their disease as a blessing, a stroke of luck, or a spiritual gift.

The Side Effects

fear	isolation
anger	frustration
anxiety	remorse
depression	guilt

How do some people, instead of hating what has happened to them, learn to embrace the experience and use it as a stepping-stone toward calmness, acceptance, and peace?

According to our experts, the power for consolation and spiritual resilience lies within us. The key to accessing your inner strength is allowing yourself the time and space necessary to acknowledge what you are feeling, understanding how these crisis-inspired emotions are affecting your life, then mindfulness/meditation/prayer, thoughtful consideration, and supportive conversation, through tapping into your own essence to uncover the well of optimism and hope that lives within each of us.

For some, this path to tranquility may be an easy, well-lit course to follow. Others may find the road fraught with dark uncertainty.

"One of the most common things my oncology patients express when we first meet is a sense of disbelief that they are having a health crisis," says psycho-oncologist Dr. Samuel Schneider. "They will say to me that 'I was feeling fine, and then suddenly a doctor looked into my eyes and told me I have a life-threatening or potentially life-ending condition.' There is a sense of incredulity about what they're hearing, a dissonance between what they feel and what their doctor says is occurring inside their bodies."

"It takes time to process the information," he continues. "It takes time to figure out, okay, what do I do now?"

In the zeal to fight back against the malignancy that has invaded our lives, many of us forget about the psychological and emotional toll disease and its treatment can have on us and those closest to us. In the quest to be well, it can be a challenge to remember that our bodies and minds are part of the same package. This connection between the physical and the psychological has to be strong and balanced if we're going to achieve integrative health.

"Very often when people are in anguish, they imagine that their release from suffering depends on a particular outcome," says Buddhist teacher and professor Kurt Spellmeyer. "But often the outcome we believe will free us occurs, and yet the problem isn't solved. We discover that it's not the situation that's making us unhappy, but rather our response to the situation."

Working toward a functional, rational response to the upheaval cancer brings to your world will have a vast, positive impact on your ability to maintain your sense of inner and outer beauty while dealing with and triumphing over this disease and its treatment. While you may be quite focused on the cellular side of your situation, don't forget to heed whatever psychological needs arise within your heart, your head, or your household. By acknowledging your fears and accepting the wildly conflicting feelings that crop up during this time, you can administer a different type of remedy to your whirling, aching mind—the healing medicine of serenity, acceptance, and peace.

WHAT'S GOING ON

Most people learning that they have a serious illness immediately begin to worry about what will happen to them and those they love. They face uncertainty about their treatment and recovery, and especially in the initial stages of a cancer diagnosis, they experience a good deal of apprehension about what this disease is going to do to their bodies and their lives.

Such reactions are perfectly normal and healthy, and they are to be expected.

But there are situations where the very word cancer sparks such intense anxiety it can easily overpower even the strongest, most positive people—fear of pain, of doctors, of needles, and of medicines; fear of the sickness itself or the loss of control it represents; fear of surgery; and fear of losing our identity, our independence, our sexuality, and our sense of self. And then of course, there is the ultimate dread: the fear of dying and the fear what may or may not await us once this earthly life is over.

While it's completely understandable for a cancer patient to experience a plethora of difficult, negative emotions when faced with this unwelcome, unwanted state of affairs, it's important to recognize that left unchecked these sentiments can drain us of the precious energy we need to become well.

"Cancer is not easy, and people looking for answers as to why this has happened may become upset to learn that the clergy doesn't have a special understanding of why an individual must face this burden," says Roman Catholic priest Father Daniel Peirano. "People want explanations. They want to be saved from their illness. They want us to pray for them, and while we do, of course, pray for their comfort, and for their souls, and for the well-being of their families, people must understand that prayer is not the only cure for illness. We must also learn to believe in medicine as an instrument of God."

Father Dan maintains that in the face of disease, the path to both physical and spiritual well-being lies along the road of appropriate medical treatment.

"You must believe that the Lord is working through your doctors, and that His blessings are revealed through science," he says. "Rather than giving in to fear and anger and all the negative emotions—rather than kneeling with your hands folded and your head bowed and expecting God to save you, you must accept the reality of your situation, and no matter how scary it is, do what you must to become well."

"We advise people not to lose hope, to continue their spiritual resistance to illness," says Muslim scholar Dr. Ahmed Nezar Kobeisy. "This includes pursuing all possible legal forms of treatment, because through science and medicine you can become closer to the truth and the light of God. By taking care of your body, you honor God's will and answer His call."

What to Do

There is no perfect recipe for maintaining your sense of spiritual beauty during cancer treatment. What resonates in one heart may leave another untouched. Allow yourself the opportunity to be honest about what you are feeling. Shutting down, isolating yourself from people who care, or drowning in denial will not improve your circumstances. A patient who is locked in resentment, buried in self-pity, or choking with fear is likely to exacerbate her condition.

If you want to cry, then cry. If you need time to be alone, make that happen. If conversation will help lighten your load, seek out a friend or a family member, call a support line, or reach out to a person of faith. Follow your instincts regarding what you need to do to cope, and don't be afraid to indulge in some necessary self-expression and examination.

While you must give expression to the full range of your feelings, temper the inclination to dwell overlong on darker thoughts.

"If you look at the whole of what needs to be done, it may seem overwhelming," says Reverend Dr. Patricia Medley, a Lutheran minister. "That's why you have to take it one day at a time. Allocate some time for the negatives, but schedule fun things too. Acknowledge your grief, but don't let it take over your life."

As a cancer survivor, Pastor Pat understands all too well how easy it can be to fall prey to disquieting thoughts and emotions.

"The thing I struggled with most is getting my sense of joy and gratitude back," she says. "It took me a long time to get through the grieving, but gradually the anger and the sorrow became smaller while other parts of my life resumed their former prominence.

"You can't let this define you," she advises. "If from the moment of diagnosis you see yourself only in terms of cancer, that becomes a terribly limiting way to go about your life."

Rabbi Jonathan Roos agrees. "In our society, people don't like you to be sad, but you have to be able to recognize and release your unhappiness in a normal, healthy way. Giving yourself permission to feel these emotions offers a great relief, but at the same time, you must make an effort to come out of the funk. As much as you're looking at your sadness, you've also got to be looking for your joy."

Kurt believes that making this effort to put your illness in perspective is central to achieving spiritual balance and physical health.

"Nothing is more important than how we approach the event itself," he says. "In Western thinking we see a separation between the body and the mind, and we look at disease as something to battle. But from the Buddhist perspective, we're not separate from the universe or the world. While we can't control the disease, we can control how we live through the experience. You can go to chemo with dread, or you can look at this as an opportunity to embrace the life you have and make it bigger, fuller, and more meaningful."

This sense of opportunity in the face of crisis isn't limited to Eastern philosophies. In fact, every religious leader we spoke with touched on this notion of perceiving cancer as not so much a catastrophe as an auspicious occasion to take the life you've lived thus far and make it resonate more richly than ever before.

"Some of us have harder loads, and we all react differently to what befalls us. In the end, we believe that illness, like everything else on this earth, comes from Allah," Sheikh Abdul Rahman Kahn says. "And though it is a test, it is also an opportunity. Looking at what comes next in your spiritual existence can be considered a chance to say things that you ought to say to those who are important to you, to put your affairs in order, to give to the poor, to right the wrongs of the past, and to make sense of the business of your life."

"God may have a plan, but we have a choice," Father Dan says. "By realizing that this earthly existence will not go on forever, you now have a new chance to be responsible for your life. God wants us to be happy, and His gift is love. If we live in His love, and express it to those around us, and take care of ourselves and our families, and do what we know in our hearts is right, that is the invitation for spiritual happiness."

Rabbi Roos concurs. "Jewish tradition is based on living life according to the laws and traditions and community and folkways of our history. The most powerful question we can ask is, How did you live your life? Were you true to yourself? Did you take care of your family and stay connected to your community? Whatever the answer, you now have the chance to embrace these concepts and live your life in a way that reflects the true essence of who you are."

"The more angry and fearful we are, the more separate we feel from what is around us," says Kurt. "But that sense of separation is an illusion and it's created by our fear. When we're unhappy and miserable and frightened, it's not just what's happening to us that's the cause, it's also how we're dealing with it.

"Traditional Western thinking is to be a fighter, to make an enemy of the situation, but I think it is more helpful to embrace the situation with a loving spirit," he says. "It is radical nonviolence. Instead of rejecting the reality of what is happening, embrace it as an experience that is part of our true being."

The idea of treating cancer as just another occurrence in our lives—no more and no less—may strike you as ridiculous or sound like a nice concept that's actually impossible to implement. But more and more doctors, hospitals, cancer centers, and support organizations recognize that a healthy spirit is integral to the overall success of our cancer care and that the effort to create a feeling of balance within our minds will have a direct, positive impact on our physical wellness.

"There is the energy of the body and the energy of the mind," says Kurt. "In the Buddhist way of thinking, these energies are fundamentally part of the same thing, so our approach is to use your body to focus your mind. If you do this—if you can learn to be receptive to the world and at one with all things—you will find the practice to be profoundly healing."

Achieving Oneness

"I'm a huge proponent of meditation," says cancer survivor and cancer specialist Dr. Leonard Wright. "We suggest it for all of our patients, and it has become so popular
here at the Wege Institute for Mind, Body and Spirit that
we now offer midday meditations once a week so that everyone can participate.

"We get a great turnout because once people understand
the benefits," he says, "they want to keep at it—patients,
doctors, nurses, and support staff. Everyone tries to attend
because it has such an incredibly freeing and empowering
impact on all of us, the caregivers as well as our patients.
It increases your energy without adding any stress to your
body or your thoughts."

Meditation is an ancient discipline that attempts to get
beyond the normal clutter of our brains by focusing the
mind on a single point of reference, be it an object, a word,
or our breath. More than 5,000 years old, the practice is a
component of almost all religions, and if done regularly
can produce a series of spiritual or psychological benefits
or both, from a higher state of consciousness and stronger
focus to greater creativity, self-awareness, or a more relaxed
and peaceful day-to-day existence.

"Everyone who is going through cancer should do meditation," Dr. Wright says. "It is a skill any patient can achieve.
If you can close your eyes and breathe and count, you can
meditate."

Dr. Wright teaches meditation to his patients in four sessions. He says the process is so simple and basic that anyone with the will to learn will quickly be able to find her own personal path to peacefulness.

"Meditative capabilities are built into each person," he says, "but this is a situation where one size fits no one. You have to find the type of meditation that works for you, be it mindfulness, mantra, relaxation, breathing, or counting. Once you demystify the process, you'll learn how to get to that peacefulness. You'll be able to control your thoughts and understand how to put stressful, negative emotions outside yourself, and that will really help you deal with your cancer more effectively."

Dr. Wright contends that meditation is essentially an intuitive practice for humans, but like most skills, it must first be learned and then maintained.

"I like to use the analogy of brushing your teeth," he continues. "You weren't born with a toothbrush in your mouth, and you needed years to get good at it, but once you became accomplished, you reaped the benefits.

"Just as you brush your teeth in the same spot and you do it at specific times of the day, I urge patients to do the same thing with meditation," Dr. Wright advises. "Establish a time and place and experiment with various techniques until you find the one that works for you."

Dr. Wright recommends *Relaxation Response* by Harvard professor Herbert Benson as an easy-to-read guide for someone who wants to understand the basics of meditation and does not have access to a teacher. Yoga centers and some health clubs offer classes in basic meditation, and video tapes and DVDs available online or from the local library can provide you with the guidance you seek.

If you are not sure if meditation is something you want to leave the house to try, there are simple ways to begin the practice right now.

Dr. Joann Weinrib, who lived in India for two years exploring Eastern medical and spiritual practices, says that taking a bit of time every day to relax and breathe will do wonders to alleviate whatever tension and anxiety is bubbling beneath your skin, and that the process is as simple as lying in bed and counting your breaths.

"It's called rhythmic breathing, and is very straightforward," she says. "You just breathe into a count, and count to specific rhythms. For instance, there is the emotional rhythm, where you breathe in for a count of six, hold the breath for a count of three, exhale for a count of six, and then hold again for another count of three.

"This exercise, done perhaps after you've awakened but before you've risen, will help lower your heart rate and center your thoughts on peaceful calm," she says. "If you keep at it and during this time try to avoid thinking of anything but counting your breath, you'll find your body falling into an amazing state of relaxation."

As a practicing Buddhist, Kurt offers another variation on finding your way to meditation.

"If you can create a unity between your body and mind, you will find it to be profoundly healing," he says. "The best time to do this is first thing in the morning. Ask the people you live with to allow you a quiet space where you can watch your breath for half an hour. Sit in a chair with a straight back. Close your eyes, and then simply breathe, a slow inhale and then a slow exhale. Focus your mind on that breath. You may count them if you like—count on the inhale, the exhale, or the absence of breath in between.

"After about fifteen minutes of concentrating on your breath, you'll find yourself starting to relax," he says. "As this happens, you'll likely find the anxieties of your life rising to the surface. They're always there, right behind the screen of your consciousness, and as you quiet your mind, you'll find them popping up.

"This is part of the meditation practice," he continues. "The mental fears and deep-seated anxieties will begin to rise to the forefront of your consciousness, and your mind will hold onto them obsessively, triggering all kinds of emotional responses.

"You may think this is getting in the way of your meditation, but it's actually part of it," he explains. "It's working through all of this; taking the time to acknowledge that the feelings exist, but then putting them outside of yourself; returning continually to the breath; remaining calm and peaceful; and allowing yourself this time every day to be relaxed and at peace.

"If you make this part of your daily life, you'll find yourself in a state of calm serenity, where your mind is really resting in the moment, and the longer you stay there, the easier it'll be to get there next time," Kurt says. "Once you achieve this state of mindful oneness, you'll find it's really quite wonderful. The thoughts or the emotional responses that were so terrifying to you earlier in your practice become more manageable. You'll be able to consider your fears and anxieties in a calmer, more serene way, and this is like medicine for your heart. It's tremendously nurturing and healing. Once you're in this state of oneness with the moment, you'll begin to feel trust in life again."

Regaining that trust in life, which can be obliterated when disease enters our personal health lexicon, can be powerfully transformative.

"Let's face it, the most horrible thing is being afraid all the time," Kurt says. "The fear of illness or death is a powerfully negative emotion that can take over our lives if we let it. That's why it's important to work on a meditative practice, to get to that place of serenely resting in the moment.

"Once you achieve this," he says, "you'll rediscover the trust you lost when you became ill. Your subconscious terrors will subside, and you'll begin to see the separation between your body and the universe as an illusion. Your body and mind will unite their energy, and you'll relax and this will help you heal."

Dr. Wright says that getting to this place of calm serenity takes a commitment, but the effort is invaluable for people with cancer. "If you get some bad news, which is not uncommon with this disease, you can rescue your day by simply putting that thought out of your mind, deciding for yourself whether you'll consider it later or just throw it away. That's a wonderful tool."

The physical benefits of meditation have been documented in medical research, which refers to the reaction as the integrative response.

As Dr. Wright explains, during meditation "you change the energy. Your CO_2 production goes way down and your oxygen consumption goes way down. Your brain waves change from delta to alpha, which are very slow and peaceful. You body's skin receptors start to change, and this is all after just five minutes."

Dr. Wright recommends all patients utilize meditation as part of their personal support efforts.

"You have to find the way to peacefulness," he says. "You have to find how to heal, and whatever is a hindrance to that should be put aside."

Thy Will Be Done

How do you create the ability to put aside the sludge that is clogging up your emotional and psychological pipes, and clear your head and your heart of draining, negative energy?

If meditation is the vehicle, then our mindset is the engine that propels us toward this necessary, empowering, and life-affirming change. Much of what happens to us during this time of illness is directly affected by how we react to the news of diagnosis and the realities of treatment. While we can't simply think, meditate, or pray our hardships away, we can work toward a greater acceptance of what's happening to us and, instead of wasting our energy locked in conflict with our current physical situation, concentrate instead on being present in the moment.

By focusing on our lives as they are actually happening and not getting caught up in a silent war within ourselves over the discomfort, pain, or unfairness that cancer represents, we enhance the overall effects of meditation by directing our energy toward physical and emotional unity, making our hearts and bodies stronger, and boosting our capacity for wellness.

Affirmation of self, maintenance of a positive outlook of

love in the face of difficulty, and a steadfast belief that no matter what happens to you, you will be okay, are essential elements of mental health and a basic tenet of almost every religion and spiritual practice humans have embraced since the beginning of consciousness. Positive thinking alleviates fear, empowers faith, and is one of the guiding principles across the spectrum of religions.

"In Christianity, they say 'Thy Will Be Done,'" says Kurt. "That spirit is the spirit of Buddhism as well. If you say thy will be done and you accept the events as they occur, then no matter what the outcome, you are all right."

Islam, too, encourages the patient to deal with health challenges in a directly spiritual way.

"Illness, though devastating, can be seen as a way for people to experience a closer relationship with God," says Dr. Kobeisy. "If you submit to God's will, if you accept, if you seek the right treatment, and if you still praise God, thank God, and appreciate the other gifts of your life, this can be a source of more blessings."

Pastor Pat believes that enlisting a higher spiritual power as a partner during treatment will strengthen your ability to heal.

"I always felt that God was my ally," she says. "When people express anger at God because they have cancer, I try to remind them that God can be an asset. With God's help we can make cancer the enemy. I look for opportunities for people to maximize their assets, and if they have significant relationships, to look at this as an opportunity to bond with and lean on those God has placed in our lives.

"You have to take the life that's given you and live it creatively," she continues. "Sure, you've been knocked down, but by accepting this event and then recovering your balance and appreciating what about your life is still good, you reject the limitations of illness and reclaim the possibilities that are still open to you."

"Give yourself the opportunity psychologically to heal the scars of illness," says Rabbi Roos. "To expand the Jewish concept to our pluralistic society, you can say you need to connect to your physical self through your community and to your spiritual self by understanding that this is not a battle with God, and there is nothing you have to do to appease or overcome God. Linking your spirituality to the sense that there is greater meaning in the world and creating a relationship with the deeper meaning is, in effect, the way to bond with God."

Even those who doubt or reject the possibility of a higher spiritual power can find solace, our experts agree, in the practice of acceptance, community, and peace.

"While you have to deal realistically with your diagnosis and whatever else is going on in your life, you also have to realize that your life can be fruitful and significant and meaningful no matter what the final outcome," Dr. Schneider says.

"The feeling of dread is like a magnet. It's like we don't ordinarily think about dying, but the minute you hear the word cancer, the sense of immortality we all have becomes interrupted, " he continues. "We have to work toward focusing not on dying but on living and on making each day as full and gratifying as it can be. Death will happen to all of us. Nothing we do can change that fact, and what's more, we really can't cross that bridge until we get there."

Today, in this moment, the only essential truth you have is the fact that you are alive. You have the ability—and it could be argued the obligation—to do what you must to enjoy the experience of life fully. In doing so, you affirm the essential point of your existence. Whether or not you attach a religious significance to the action, you bond with what clergy believe is the presence of the greater powers of the universe within you.

"Dying is part of being mortal," says Pastor Pat. "The last time I checked, the mortality rate among humans was still one hundred percent. We don't usually dwell on that fact when we're healthy. But if in the midst of dealing with cancer we decide to concentrate on making memories with those we love and continue to live creatively and well, it's a sort of defiance, a creative defiance to resolve that you're going to live as well as you possibly can and let death come whenever its time has arrived."

"To be fully present in the moment is so potent and powerfully beautiful," says Kurt. "If you can find a way to the oneness, then the guilt, the fear, the anxiety, the depression—all these problems—are all solved because death ceases to be a reality at all. It's just a change of form.

"You can imagine yourself as a wave in the ocean," he says. "You exist as a person. You are real, and as with the wave, for a little while you are separate from the larger body of water, but eventually the wave ends. It recedes and returns to the ocean of life.

"If you are the wave, you are separate from the greater ocean, but only for a relatively short period of time; you are still water, and when you return to the ocean, you are returning to the source from which you came. Now, expanding the thought further, you can see that new waves are constantly forming, and rising, and folding back into the ocean, but that the ocean is always there. This is a metaphor for your true self. You really are part of the universe, the universe is infinite, and so no matter where in the cycle you are, you are still part of the whole, and in this way you can never truly die."

The Muslim concept of eternal existence is similar, though expressed in a different way, as Sheikh Rahman explains.

"Life is a circle," he says. "You go from your time with God in pre-birth to your life, your grave, and then your afterlife when you return to the circle of God. It's all about returning back to the truth and the light and the peace that is Allah. It's all about recognizing that life is fragile, and we should do what we must to ensure that our soul and spirit are ready for this return. That is why when someone dies we say, 'From Allah we have come and unto Him is our return.'"

"Life is not ended by death," Dr. Kobeisy concurs. "Death is another form of life, and so there is nothing to fear."

The power to be happy, and peaceful, and fully engaged in our lives rests exclusively inside of us and can be best expressed by reaching out to those in our path for support and guidance and love.

"If you depend only on God, you are denying the actual

presence of God in the other people He has put into your life," Father Dan says. "You must be open to touch, to conversation, and to the plans of others because God reveals Himself in those who are close to us on this earth. Denying this is to deny the action of God in your life, whereas accepting this initiates healing."

"People are all the same no matter where they come from or what they believe," Sheikh Rahman says. "We all want to be happy and healthy and to have our families near us. We want security and comfort. What brings us together as human beings is far stronger than what separates us. Instead of questioning or lamenting what befalls us, it is better to surrender to what has happened, find the joy that remains in your soul, and then pursue what you must to rebuild your health, and your spirit, and your life."

Rather than spending precious energy wrestling with the "why" of your condition, our experts agree that a much more useful expenditure of time is to eliminate the question, since it has no answer, and resolve to make the most of the life, the circumstances, and the relationships you have on this day, in this moment, with this breath.

When you find your attitude is sometimes less than inspirational, you can take solace in the fact that your negativity, too, is perfectly fine.

"You can be pissed off about what's happening to you," Dr. Schneider says. "Being down won't affect your prognosis or harm your condition. But if you give yourself the space to enjoy the gamut of other, more fruitful emotions that will come to you, you'll have a more optimistic outlook and a better day.

"Latch onto life," he advises. "It's useless to focus on death or to feel guilty because you're not upbeat and happy on any given day. You're not going to deteriorate by admitting you're angry about having cancer. But if you keep your mind on what really matters to you in this life, all the other elements will fall into place, and you may find yourself coming out of this experience more positive and hopeful than you ever were before."

Crisis = Opportunity

In their written language, some interpret the Chinese symbol for crisis as a symbol that also suggests opportunity. There is certainly a pronounced possibility of harvesting great opportunity in the crisis of cancer, if the patient is willing to look beyond the immediate fear and turmoil of her diagnosis and see the potential to create a fuller, more meaningful life.

"In Islam, we believe that an illness such as cancer can be seen as a gift because you now have the chance to improve your life in an effort to please God," Dr. Kobeisy says. "You now have the opportunity to correct whatever victims may have been hurt as a result of your own sin—to do good deeds, to help the poor and disadvantaged, and to affirm your love for your family.

"Having this condition also enables you to become a role model for humanity, through your patience, your perseverance, and your dedication to becoming well," he adds.

Dr. Schneider agrees that while initially devastating, cancer can represent a way for you to become closer to being the person you have always wanted to be.

"Patients often feel like they're a passenger in a car that is careening out of control and they have to depend on others to bring that car under control," he says. "The feeling of being subject to the whims and decisions of others creates a tremendous sense of loss and can lead to anger and frustration."

The remedy he says is in being honest about what you are going through and in using this experience to open doors to a deeper relationship with those who are close to you.

"Have that open dialogue to admit that what is happening to you is not normal. Be willing not only to express what you are feeling and thinking, but also to allow others to express their own thoughts and feelings to you," Dr. Schneider says. "If you invite the conversation and are willing to both express your truths and listen to another person's, then the attachment you share will be stronger. There will be an enhanced sense of getting through the experience together, and the result will be a much stronger bond and an improved ability to communicate."

"If you go back to the wave analogy," says Kurt, "you could say that this is part of the adventure of being alive, another challenge to face as we pull our energy from the ocean to create our fleeting individuality. If we approach cancer in that spirit, as an invitation to embrace whatever it is life throws our way and make the most of it, then it's impossible to lose."

"What I learned from cancer is that you only have so

much physical life," Pastor Pat says. "With the time you have on this earth, you can do things that are far more significant than perhaps you were doing before. I think there's nothing like a good scare to help you prioritize what is important in your life."

If there is a friend you have been meaning to reach out to, a relative you would like to be closer with, a child who should know you better, or a neighbor who might benefit from something you know or could do, now is the time to act. By reaching out to the people in your family, your social circle, and your community, you align yourself with the living, breathing energy of everyone around you, and the resulting influx of care, appreciation, stimulation, and satisfaction will help you move through the days of your treatment.

A Family Affair

The devastation of illness directly affects those closest to us. Spouses, children, parents, siblings, friends, and extended family all feel the impact of the diagnosis. They too must learn to cope with the changes, both physical and emotional, that cancer brings.

"Much of what you are in sickness is about who you were when you were well," says Rabbi Roos. "While you can't take away the grief people will face when they learn you are ill, there is much you can do to make it easier on them and yourself."

Putting together the business of your life, as Sheikh Rahman calls it, should be one of your first priorities. "You cannot take away another's pain. You cannot personally remove their sadness," he says. "But you can act in a way that affirms your essential goodness. You can express your love, your hopes, and your dreams for them. You can show them through your actions how you want them to behave. And you can leave a legacy of faith and acceptance that will inspire those with you now and those yet to come."

Dr. Schneider maintains that putting things to right will settle the spirit and make you feel better as well. "I find that if you have completed your will, designated a health proxy, signed a living will, made arrangements for power of attorney and property disbursements, and the like, it's very useful. It creates a sense of control that these important issues have been taken care of.

"But it goes further," he adds. "Writing letters, saying what needs to be said, gathering people together to tell them what they need to hear—these things all contribute to your sense of completeness, of doing the right thing, and of creating a legacy that those who love you will always be able to hold close."

If you're at a loss as to how to begin such a process, consider writing an ethical will, which is essentially a letter to your family, friends, and community that shares your values, your dreams, and the lessons you have learned over the course of your life.

"I'm a big proponent of ethical wills," says Rabbi Roos. "As living creatures, we are so much more than the assets we have collected. This is a way to ensure that the spiritual, intangible side of you is as well disseminated as your material possessions."

While they have no legal standing, ethical wills can often become priceless documents for you and those who love you.

"It's such an important process for many people to work out," Rabbi Roos continues. "Once you begin, you're essentially composing a narrative of how you want your life to be viewed and remembered, which inspires many questions along the lines of what you want your spouse, your children, your friends, and your siblings to know about you. It's a great way to take stock of your life, your values, and your choices and write them down for posterity."

Like a telegram to the future, an ethical will can project all your dreams and desires, visions and values, passions and ponderings into a world yet to come, giving those you care for, those who may not yet be old enough to understand, and even those not yet born a tangible sense of your personality, and perhaps even your soul, through your presentation of words, pictures, songs, and creative collections.

"You can start with a blank page or use a template from the Internet," Rabbi Roos suggests. "You can clip out articles that resonate for you and put them in a folder, or list the books, songs, or paintings that inspired you. You can make voice recordings or video recordings. It's really about creating a testament to your values, which you can then pass along, and these become so dear. It is as if your voice and your face and your heart remain with the living for all time."

"It's very useful to consider what you want people to know about you," Dr. Schneider says, "because it gives you a deeper understanding of yourself. These exercises in communication go far to make patients feel like the loose ends are tied and things have been made right. This all helps create a feeling of calm, of being settled, as well as creating the satisfied feeling that comes from doing the right thing. You're more complete."

Ethical wills are an ancient tradition practiced at one point or another by almost every culture on the planet. While they began many thousands of years ago as oral presentations, composing a modern document can begin at any point in a person's life and be revised or updated as the years go by. The value they bring to a person facing illness is a sense of closure, of being settled and of having effectively communicated what is most important in your life to those who are most important to you.

Atlas in a Skirt

Despite the mythological image of the world balanced on a large man's shoulders, women are usually the foundation of their worlds, holding up their families, their children, their homes, and their businesses, all at once. During illness, the burden may become too great, and our shoulders might sag. Those who depend on us for the million things we do may become a bit resentful that we're not able to fulfill our roles with the same vigor and flair we've always had. They may become angry or depressed. And so, for that matter, might we.

Outside help, in the form of clergy, therapy, or support groups or all three, may offer their own little bit of personal salvation for an individual or family in need.

"It was once hard for me to speak with people who were suffering because I thought they expected me to have the answers for them, and I didn't have any," Father Dan says. "But what I learned is that it's really about listening. People want to be listened to. They want to be heard. They want to know someone cares.

"By giving people a safe place to speak about whatever is on their minds, I help them find peace," he continues. "We pray for their family and their kids, and they come to understand that even in dark times, they are not alone. God is close and they receive a wonderful gift of serenity and understanding. And I am blessed as well. When I leave them, I am filled with hope."

"One of my jobs as a member of the clergy is to help people through an emotionally difficult set of circumstances a loved one may not be able to deal with," Rabbi Roos says. "It goes beyond denomination. If you reach out, it doesn't matter which faith you first touch, you'll find someone whose mission is to help you."

Hospital chaplains are trained to minister to all patients regardless of their religious affiliations. They can be a great starting point in locating a spiritual representative to help you through your more difficult times. They also are dedicated patient advocates who will help you should you need special assistance with nurses, doctors, food services, or anything else that happens while you are in the hospital. You can speak with the chaplain about psycho-oncologists, therapists, and support groups, and they will do all they can to connect you to the people who can be of the most help.

"Most major medical centers will have psychiatrists and psychologists on staff who are trained to deal with people with a cancer diagnosis," Dr. Schneider says. "If you find yourself unable to cope with your thoughts or feelings, if you're losing your passion for life or the things that once pleased you, it may be time to reach out to a professional who can help you manage whatever you're facing."

You can call the referral desk of the closest major medical center, even if you're not being admitted, and get a list of accredited doctors who are well versed in cancer and its impact on the mind and spirit. Speak with a few, until you find one with whom you feel at ease and able to express yourself.

"Oftentimes, patients will be very reluctant to talk with family members about how they're feeling because they don't want them to be even more worried or put a larger burden on their shoulders," Dr. Schneider explains. "Talking with someone who's neutral, who isn't emotionally vested in you, can be quite cathartic and healing."

The same can be said for those in your circle who are not managing your situation in a healthy way. Children especially may need some outside assistance as they try to work through their own disappointments or anxieties about what is happening to you.

Your oncologist may be the best person to ask where to turn for help should you or someone you care for need support. Because of that person's intimate knowledge of your condition and the trust you have in that person's care, that doctor is often able to recommend where you might turn for a helping hand. If you find that you or someone important to you is falling into what may be clinical depression, it is imperative to speak with a doctor who can prescribe ways to alleviate the condition.

"It's very important for individuals to recognize depression and to seek appropriate treatment," Dr. Kobeisy says. "People who are withdrawn or isolated or depressed won't respond as they should to their cancer treatment. They must be cared for if they are to heal."

"Changes in the way people usually function are a significant clue that intervention may be required," Dr. Schneider says. "If you find that you or someone close to you is apathetic, has lost interest in gardening or cooking or any of the things that once were a source of great pleasure, it's important to get them engaged, to talk with them, and to find out what's going on."

"The second indicator is severe personality changes. If someone suddenly becomes excessively irritable or grumpy or nervous or tearful, these are signs that there's too much being buried, and there needs to be an opening up."

Both patients and those they love walk a fine line in terms of how and when to intervene.

"Denial is a pretty good defense mechanism," Dr. Schneider explains. "It's not a good idea to interfere with this because it's one of the ways people monitor their own reactions and maintain a sense of optimism. As long as there's an underlying understanding of the situation and there aren't any debilitating or self-destructive behaviors going on—you know, refusing treatment or never getting out of bed or not being able to stop crying—I think it's best to let things be."

If a doctor or support person recommends some anti-depressive drugs, don't panic about putting more medications into your system. Short-term fixes can help you through a rough patch, and as soon as you are in a better place, your need for them will end.

"As you get back on your feet, you'll wean off these drugs," Dr. Schneider says. "Just like the treatment and the side effects, this medication is only temporary."

But I'm Still Bald . . .

Anything that detracts from our appearance takes a toll on our psyches, especially as treatment goes on and the punishing nature of the medications continues to reveal itself on our outer shell.

Despite our best efforts to look as well as we can, some people might still notice something is amiss. They may not be as kind or discreet with their reactions as we might like. The ability to see through the less-than-stellar behavior of others and the power to make the most of what we've got lies within us.

"Paul talks about this in the Bible, where he says, 'While our bodies are wasting our spirits are being renewed every day,'" Pastor Pat says. "Your physical body may not be what you're accustomed to, but in wisdom and self-acceptance, you should be growing more and more beautiful every day.

Your spiritual self becomes brighter and more luminous every time you answer the questions, how can I be more loving, more hopeful, or more helpful as a guide to others through my experience?"

"The Prophet says beauty does not look at your face, nor your wealth, but your heart and actions," Sheikh Rahman says. "If you are interested in being a good human being, then beauty is not particularly useful, especially if it is all in your hair and not in your heart."

"If you are comfortable with your own values and culture and believe you are living a good human experience, you are far more beautiful than someone who compares you against a socially constructed concept that does not reflect the beauty of the spirit," Dr. Kobeisy says.

Even as you search for hair, makeup, and clothing choices that make you comfortable, you may find yourself struggling to accept the changes to your physical appearance.

"I've met many women who have a hard time looking at themselves during and right after treatment because they can't accept what the disease and the surgery and the chemo have done to their bodies," Dr. Schneider says. "To counteract these issues, I remind them that this was something that happened to them. It wasn't their fault, and while they may not have any control over the medical process, they can control how they react to their body problems. They can be in the driver's seat when it comes to making decisions about what they can do to look and feel better."

No matter how your appearance changes during your treatment, when the cosmetics are washed away and the hairpiece is in the closet, your beauty remains because it emanates from inside you.

"Human beings pay attention to how they're being judged by others on the basis of how they look. It's as true for men as it is for women. My response is, it doesn't matter how other people see you," Dr. Kobeisy says. "What matters is, how do you appear in the sight of God? Are you a good and decent person? Do you feel you reflect God's will? If your answer to these questions is yes, then anyone who does not recognize the beauty of your soul is not worthy of your friendship or acquaintance."

"In these struggles, I think the principle of not separating yourself from a community of survivors is very important because you become part of a larger entity, the entity of women helping women, and you can speak with them in ways that will inspire empathy as well as sympathy," Rabbi Roos says. "Among these people, you can discuss things that may seem unimportant to those not dealing with cancer, including how you feel about your looks, and there won't be any discomfort because you're all essentially speaking the same language, feeling the same feelings. You can help not only yourself but others in the group who are facing similar difficulties."

"There are hundreds of thousands of people on this planet who are physically beautiful but spiritually vicious," Sheikh Rahman says. "Once you realize how shallow the concept is, you must come back to yourself and appreciate your self-perception. This is really all we have. This is what we take with us when the circle of life returns us to heaven."

The Quiet Hours

During your cancer experience, there will be times when you will be by yourself. You may awaken during the night feeling tense. A hoped-for nap may become elusive after some disturbing news, a reaction to the chemo may make you feel ill, or you may find you cannot turn off the voices in your head.

Meditation is helpful. Exercise will also ease your mind. And twenty-four-hour support centers can provide a lifeline of understanding when no one else is around.

You may also wish for some solace from saints and prophets and scholars whose wisdom continues to resonate long after they have died. Luckily, you can choose from many texts: the Torah, the Bible, the Koran and the Sacred Texts of the Buddha are just the beginning of a library that reflects the deep thoughts, poems, and prayers of humanity, from the Book of David and the Beatitudes to the poetry of Walt Whitman and the teachings of Mother Teresa.

"I am a person of the Word, and I had a real reliance on scripture, not in terms of rigorous practice, but just comfort and inspiration," Pastor Pat says. "For instance, when I went for the mammography that first identified my cancer, I knew from the amount of times I had to go back for more pictures that something was wrong. I was growing more and more frightened. What came to me was, "Keep me as the apple of your eye. Hide me under the shelter of your wings" (Psalm 117), and this became a theme for me. I felt near to God's breast and God's heart. Birds appeared whenever I was facing a difficult moment, and it seemed as if God were sending me the message that the Holy Spirit, who is often represented as a dove, was near. And this gave me great comfort."

"Going back to the ancient texts and discovering that an ancestor three thousand years ago faced something similar to what you're going through reminds you that in your suffering you aren't alone in the scope of human history," Rabbi Roos says. "You may read the Psalms or the older stories; you may pick up a book of prayer or meditation and find a message that works for you. That's why I recommend that people have a compilation of inspirational writings so that they can browse through the sayings until they find the one that brings them solace. It doesn't matter where it comes from. You can be Jewish and find great meaning in the words of a Hindu philosopher. Have a personal prayer that is relevant to you so that during those times when you're not with your doctor, or your therapist, or your clergy, or your friend, you can remember your prayer and find consolation in that."

If after reading or searching online you cannot find an already written piece that resonates for you, make one up yourself. It doesn't matter what the words are, as long as the message eases your mind and brings you a sense of peace.

The Prayer of Life

Faith is a very personal matter. No one can instill in your heart the tranquility of a monk or the dedication of a missionary. Whatever you believe is for you to decide, and whatever brings you the sense of purpose and resolve you need to get through cancer is undoubtedly the right thing for you.

But while arguments regarding the existence of God and heaven and the concepts of sin and redemption are unlikely to be resolved anytime soon, one thing all people can unify around is our passion for life and our desire to keep it for as long as our bodies will allow.

Being alive is a blessing. Being human is a gift, a celebration, a joy, and a wonder. Regardless of how we may have felt before diagnosis, once we realize that our existence in this time and space is only temporary, grabbing onto the energy that fills your body and doing everything we can to preserve and enhance it must be our top priority.

"I think it's kind of comforting that we're all living the same kind of experience and that we have this commonality that all living things must go through, which is birth and life and death. No one is exempt," Pastor Pat says. "But I believe God is there for all of us, and even if you don't embrace all the tenets of your faith, as Martin Luther says, 'It's the mutual consolation of the brethren.' You need to break away from the isolation of our times, and whether or not you have the faith you need, you can still find solace and comfort in a worshipping community. If you come to a service, you will be part of something bigger than yourself, and you will always be welcome."

"Being connected to your community, whether it's a community of faith or family or friends, provides you with the opportunity to heal psychologically," Rabbi Roos says. "But it also represents a responsibility on your part to return to the community the energy they gave to you. You must engage with the world, and continue to take care of your body, and live your life in the way that reflects your true self."

Father Dan says that our chance for experiencing the joys of heaven is before us each and every day of our lives.

"If my life here on earth is hell and I have no love and I have no happiness, then my afterlife will be that same hell, because there is no difference spiritually. We are creating what will come next, and in this life, if we answer God's call to love ourselves and our neighbors, to care for our children and our world, and to be truthful and giving and decent, then we are in heaven right now."

Spirituality and psychological health do not come from a building or a series of words or a pill. It's not about reciting a bunch of lines from a text. It's about understanding the words, internalizing them, and acting on them.

If we can find within ourselves the power to be at peace, the will to accept our situation, and the strength to trust in our worth, then nothing that happens to our bodies can ever truly weaken us.

That is the prayer we offer. That is the blessing we seek. It may or it may not exist on some plane, but for those who are willing to dedicate themselves to that holy place within, where all is calm and tranquil, they will find an undeniable truth: that heaven is a place on earth.

For more information on the topics discussed in this chapter, please type one of these phrases into your search bar:

Ethical Wills

Living Wills

Health Care Proxy

Last Will and Testament

Inspirational Writings

Spiritual Writings

Religious Writings

Meditation

Or visit the following sites:

www.ethicalwill.com

www.freeethicalwill.com

www.wise4living.com

www.caringinfo.org

www.uslivingwillregistry.com

www.theosophy.com

www.angel.com

www.allspirit.co.uk

www.isna.net

www.icofa.com

www.religioustolerance.org

www.jewfaq.com

Parting Pearls

"BC" has many different meanings in this world. It can stand for "Before Christ," "Before College," or "Before Children." But once you've been diagnosed, your world will always be divided into two distinct phases—"Before Cancer" and everything that comes after.

Hard as it may seem to believe right now, once your treatment ends, life will return to normal. Eventually, you'll pass whole chunks of time without giving a single thought to cancer. But the memory of what you faced will remain inside you and, in a variety of ways both large and small, change you forever.

As you move through your cancer journey, our experts and survivors have each expressed a wish for you. Consider these their parting bits of wisdom from people you may never meet, but who want you to know that you are braver than you think, smarter than you know, and more beautiful than you could ever imagine.

From Marybeth

About two years after I completed chemo, an article in *The New York Times* got me thinking about the changes cancer and chemotherapy had on me. Called "Is Looking Your Age the New Taboo?" it reported that Americans were so afraid of showing their age that women who had yet to turn 30 were undergoing plastic surgery to reverse what they feared was their loss of youthful beauty.

This message really hit a nerve with me because "BC" I was one of those women, always fighting the battle against gravity, cellulite, and wrinkles. When cancer came knocking, I finally stopped worrying about being super fit and shiny and smooth and learned to cut myself a break. I wrote this letter to the editor of *The New York Times*, which was published a few days later:

"Who's the Youngest of Them All?"

Published: March 5, 2007
To the Editor:
Long before sunscreen was a standard ingredient in moisturizer, I stayed out of the sun. I exercised, did yoga, ate grains, avoided meat, colored my hair and maintained a body mass index of 18. Though I loved it when people thought I was a decade younger than my actual age, I never for one moment relaxed in my battle against aging.

Then I was diagnosed with cancer. My breasts were removed. My hair fell out. My once-perfect skin was scarred from surgery, my formerly limber joints creaked, my rosy skin turned sallow and steroids included in my chemotherapy shot my weight up 20 pounds.

Today, at 46, I'm in menopause. I carry an extra 10

pounds that just won't go away. I have wrinkles, graying
hair and limited flexibility. I also have a profound sense
of my "real" beauty. Where I once sought perfection, I now
celebrate my life, and my triumph over disease gives me
a beauty no cream or vial can provide.

I once believed that I'd be going for injections to smooth
those lines around my mouth and brow. But now I'm
proud to look my age; I've earned every year.

My hope is that you'll be proud of what you've done to
fight your disease. You've earned the right to stand tall no
matter what sickness has done to your body. Don't believe
for a second you aren't gorgeous because anyone who can
do what we have, look cancer in the eye and refuse to blink,
is truly, deeply, spiritually beautiful.

From Debbie

Remember to ask for support. Those around you may
be just as afraid, or even more afraid, than you are. Reach
out and you'll find the comfort you may seek. Be strong,
but don't go it alone. Those who love and care will be there
so that together you can make the journey toward recovery.

From Ahmed Nezar Kobeisy, Ph.D.

There are the illnesses of the physical body and the illnesses of the soul, the heart, and the mind. If we have health
in our souls and our minds and our hearts, we are much
better off than those who have physical health but are spiritually ill. See the work of Allah in the medical treatments
you receive, and use your illness to take you higher in your
faith. If you can do this, you will find hope, strength, per-

severance, and courage. You will become closer to the peace and beauty of God.

From Amy Gibson

Who we are is the essence of what we carry. No one can take that from us. You can lose your hair, but you'll never lose your essence. So put your makeup on and go to chemo dressed like the lady you are. Believe in yourself and try not to give into depression or think of yourself as sick. The better you feel about yourself when dealing with a health issue, the greater your success will be.

From Amy Bragagnini

In the big picture of your life, this is a speed bump, not a roadblock. Get your treatment, whatever that entails, and then move on. Enlist all the help that's available for you, from dietitians to support groups to exercise and spiritual care. Get whatever you need to be well in both body and spirit.

From Anastasia

Be strong, and believe and feel with your entire body that you will overcome this. Our bodies react amazingly to our emotions, so remember to keep positive.

From Betsey

Don't be afraid to talk about it. Open up to your closest supporters and make a plan for how you're going to deal with this time. Let them help you stay focused on what you need to do. Don't forget the support groups. There's such a community out there, such a sisterhood that you can be part of—it's really amazing!

From Brian Torpey, M.D.

Medicine is constantly changing and doctors now are far more approachable than they once were, so don't hesitate to ask questions. Take advantage of information technology to learn what you can about your condition, what's going on, and what you're dealing with. Tap into all the positive support that's out there, so you have whatever you want and need to get through this.

From Cheryl

You always need someone to talk to, so find a counselor or someone to confide in, talk with, and cry with. Women don't do well at asking for things. You have to learn to let go of that and ask for what you need. Do research. Make sure you understand what you're being told, and don't be afraid to speak up if there's something you don't understand. Upset the applecart if it's in your best interest to do this, and put yourself first whenever you can.

From Chris

Positive thinking is essential to recovery. You just have to focus on life and on all that you still want to accomplish. Let that be your inspiration. No matter how hard it is for you, others have faced even greater difficulties. If they can do it, so can you.

From Christine

I've never met a woman who loved everything about her body. The whole point of fashion is to make the most of what you've got. If you want, you can look stylish every day. This situation is only temporary. Embrace the new you and look forward to getting better.

From Deann

Find the friends who will be strong with you, and let them help you. It is not easy to lose your hair, but if you have the support you need, it will be a lot less traumatic to experience these side effects. If you open yourself up to people, you will find that there are many who want to lend you a hand.

From Eivind

Be an advocate for yourself. Do what you must to find the answers you seek and do not be afraid. Be kind. Be strong. Find uplifting friends. Lean on a strong shoulder, stay busy, and live your life with optimism, as close to normal as you can.

From Father Dan

We are all joined in the long line of life. It is not only us, it is all creation, all the people who ever were or ever will be who share God's presence and enjoy God's salvation. No one is ever alone. God is always with us.

From Francine

I believe in hope, but hope alone doesn't get you anywhere. Combine hope with passion—for your life, your health, your family, for the things that really matter to you—and that will get you through. Focus on the passions that resonate in your soul and you will heal. Your future will once again be what you want it to be.

From Gayle

Women don't ordinarily put themselves first or allow themselves to be taken care of, so when help is offered, say yes. Throw out everything in your life that you don't need and isn't working. Draining friends, needing to have your house spotless, being president of the PTA—if it's too much for you, let it go, and concentrate on what works for you and makes you calm and relaxed and happy.

From Howard Murad, M.D.

Isolation is prevalent in our society for both the healthy and the sick. My advice is to reduce that isolation because when you are ill it is common to withdraw from others. At the same time it is vital to acknowledge your feelings. Join a support group or network where you can openly discuss what is going on psychologically and emotionally. I believe you will be healthier and stronger if you do.

From Joann Weinrib, Chiropractor

Keep the faith. You're on a journey now that will change your life. All the people I know who have gone through this have come out of it much stronger. Now you'll have a new life story. Trust that your inner strength will help you do whatever you need to be well.

From John

Have faith. It is our greatest ally when faced with adversity and fear. Let go of fear, which is our biggest nemesis and can undermine our ability to aid ourselves in the healing process. Love is life's most powerful force. When we call on it and collectively use it for a given task, we can conquer suffering. Smile and laugh as much as you can, for they are two of the best remedies for healing almost any affliction.

From Krista

I know what you have to face will not be easy, but you are not alone, and there is nothing wrong with wanting to look good. Of course, beauty starts from within. During this time, if you can look in the mirror and be happy with what you see, that will boost your endorphins, which are nature's high, and they in turn will boost your immune system. Go ahead and pamper yourself—by looking better, you will not only feel better, but you will actually help your body heal.

From Leonard Wright, M.D.

Look at yourself and understand why you want to live and then use that as your anchor to this world. Make your reasons part of your fiber and your soul, and fit this motivation into every part of your life. Envision your future, and make plans for it so that you are always moving toward your dreams and goals.

From Lloyd Gayle, M.D.

Take it one day at a time. Deal with each issue and symptom as it comes. Don't try to prejudge things and don't try to anticipate what's going to happen next, just go with what's happening and know it will be over. It *will* end.

From Kurt

You are part of the universe, not separate from it. If you make trust your path and embrace your illness as part of yourself, you may find that what is happening to you will help you wake up to the oneness of everything, and through that you will find your true nature. Look at this experience as a challenge to be spiritually at peace, and embrace this opportunity to find serenity and calm. If you can find your way to the oneness of everything, then nothing bad will ever happen. No matter what occurs, it is all good.

From Leah

Do whatever you need to do to look good, or hot, or make you feel your best. A lot of this is internal—the strength and the bravery and the fight to be well. Be strong and be positive. Even if we don't know you personally, we're still pulling for you. The world is on your side.

From Louis Philippe

We are social beings. You can't become a recluse and close the doors. Get out there and talk to people so that you know you're not alone. Focus on what you can do to feel better about yourself. It's a bit of a process, but this is not the end. There's so much help and more and more people are surviving. It's like HIV—once that meant life was over, but now it's just an illness you live with. Make a plan, like a recipe, and then follow it through.

From Michele

This is just a transitory moment in time. It will pass, so don't hide under a bush and fear the changes that have occurred. Concentrate on how you are going to feel your best during this phase of your life. Your future is coming. Hang onto hope and deal with what is happening as best you can so that you still get out there every day and live your life to the fullest.

From Noah Gilson, M.D.

The benefits of treatment far outweigh the difficulties. The side effects will fade over time. Hang in there and trust that, though it is tough, the chemo will work and you will be okay.

From the Oncology Nurses at Princeton Medical Group

People want to be supportive. Accept every bit of help that is offered to you. Line up people to drive you to your chemo, or take notes for you at your doctor's visits, or prepare some meals, or keep an eye on your kids. Be honest with them about what you need. You'll find caring volunteers ready to be of service to help you get through.

From Oribe

It's important to keep a good head throughout this whole thing, and find ways to make yourself look attractive. You need confidence and courage. Be strong and brave and if you can, keep a sense of humor. Someday you'll laugh about when you had to shave your head.

From Oscar

Look ahead to the future and keep a positive spirit. You are not alone and there is a light at the end of the tunnel. As time goes by you will grow healthy and strong, and so will your hair.

From Pastor Pat

What is impossible for human beings is possible through God. Be kind to yourself. Take it one day at a time, one task at a time. Decide what you need to do today and then just do that one thing. Lean on your friends. Don't be afraid or ashamed to feel grief, or anger, or anything negative. You can't choose your feelings—if you try, you do violence to the way God made you. You can't tune out the negative, because then the positive feelings are not happening naturally, either. Just accept that this is happening to you, that it is part of life, and that it will pass. God is with you. Find strength through faith.

From Patricia

Think positive. Be your own advocate; stay on top of the literature. Fear only decreases as time passes and when you are feeling well. Accept help—most people want to help and are kind. Be selfish—put your needs first. Give your body what it needs to heal.

From Patricia Wexler, M.D.

Wanting to look good is not trivial. It's about you feeling healthy and good about yourself. It's not about just being grateful that you're alive; it's about being grateful that you're alive and also facing every day with your best foot, and your best attitude, forward. You don't have to present yourself to the world looking sick. You can feel healthy, you can look healthy, and you can be healthy. When I see my patients embrace this attitude, it makes me very happy.

From Peter Staats, M.D.

There are a lot of options for patients today, so don't suffer silently. If you're in pain or you're uncomfortable, search for ways to be better. Speak to different doctors, look for different treatments, and don't stop until you find what you need. Don't settle, and don't take no for an answer.

From Rabbi Roos

Don't lose sight of who you've been your entire life until this moment of diagnosis, and be that person. Stay true to who you are, to your real self, and don't let this change how you see yourself. Be the person you've always been, and continue to strive to be the person you want to be.

From Rick

Don't compare or anticipate what is going to happen to you based on someone else's experience. You'll have your own journey, and it'll be as individual as you are, so don't get caught up in celebrity stories or movies or in what others say is the right thing to do. Follow your own instincts and deal with the changes that are happening to you as best you can. It's okay to want to look good, and when you do, you'll feel better.

From Robert

I do not recommend that women who are ill or going through chemotherapy try to disguise themselves with layers of glamour. Instead, wear what consoles you and is in tune with your inner feelings. As a patient faces fears of all kinds, it is most important to get yourself grounded into a more pure state of consciousness so that you can see the inner light of God and know that angels are all around, watching over you.

From Rosemarie

Take full advantage of your support system. It's important to have people around you who'll listen if you want to talk and let you be quiet if that's your preference. I tried to shut people out because I didn't understand how much they cared. If I had one thing I could change about that time, it would be to open up to those who wanted to help me and let them be there for me. It's important to make yourself participate in the world even if you want to be private about your illness. If you do, you'll find that you're really not alone.

From Samuel Schneider, Ph.D.

Depend on those who love you and who will be there for you, and do whatever you need. Don't be afraid to speak about your feelings, and let those who care express theirs to you. Let people know if they're doing too much or being overbearing. It's perfectly natural to want space, or feel bad, or wish for solitude. People will be there to help you, as long as you let them know both what you need and what you don't.

From Sandy Canzone, O.M.D.

You're not a statistic. The body wants to live, and you can give it that chance. If there's a friend or anyone who'll walk this walk with you, let them. You aren't alone.

From Sheikh Rahman

See this moment as an opportunity to increase your faith, and take the life that is still yours and use it very well. Use your illness as a blessing for all those who know you, who interact with you, and who love you. Your positive approach to your illness may give you so much strength that what you have put off and pretended to ignore your entire life will be understood and made right. Through this, you will see the work of Allah in our lives. Use it to be well.

From Theresa

This disease will run its course. It does not change who you are. This is a temporary setback. Embrace how you look, and do what you can to make it better. Handle this with the dignity and respect you are due. Make yourself look as beautiful and feel as beautiful as you can, and when this is over, you will be empowered and more beautiful than you ever thought you could be.

From Thomas A. Caputo, M.D.

Be strong. You are not the first to have to face this and you will not be the last, but you will be well again. Just reach into yourself and find the courage, and the will, to do whatever you need to make it through.

ACKNOWLEDGMENTS

If learning you've got cancer is one of those life experiences that prove how much people need the support of family, friends, and community, as authors we found that writing a book about cancer treatment is surely another.

While we created this book, we know that without the help of the following people we would not have been able to generate a single word. So with the deepest gratitude we thank all the experts who participated in this project and gave so willingly of their time, expertise, and experience. Thanks as well to their assistants and support staff who worked tirelessly to make sure that the interviews took place, that the quotes were verified, and that every deadline was met.

We also send our heartfelt thanks and warmest regards to survivors Chris, Laura, Patricia, and Rosemarie for sharing the intimate details of their cancer experiences to inspire chemo girls everywhere.

Very special thanks to Betsey Johnson for sharing her

257

energy, her enthusiasm, and her amazing spirit and for contributing a fantastic foreword. Thanks to Agatha Sczcepaniak for working so hard to pull it all together.

Heartfelt thanks to Dan Brestle, vice chairman and president of the Estée Lauder Companies, North America, and Donna Rapisarda for recognizing early on the importance of our project and putting us in touch with so many wonderful experts; to LouAnne Rourke of the Personal Care Products Council and Lisa Burris at The Look Good Feel Better Foundation® for coordinating our interviews with their specialists in hair, wigs, skin care, and makeup; and to Pauline Brown, board member of the Avon Foundation, for her insight, advice, and ever-ready support.

Great thanks to our agent, Anne Hawkins of John Hawkins and Associates, and her colleague Moses Cardona for "getting" our book the moment they received our proposal and connecting us with Michaela Hamilton at Kensington Books, who enthusiastically embraced our work and gave *Beauty Pearls* its home.

A big hug and thank you to attorney Stacy Kohn, who gives new meaning to the practice of seamlessly combining business and friendship with such dedication and flair.

Warmest appreciation to Krista Dibsie, Carla Scarabino, and Jacqueline Tobacco at the Beauty Foundation for Women's Cancer Care for their enthusiasm and support for our book and for their ongoing commitment to doing all they can to improve the lives of women facing cancer treatment. Thanks as well to Michele McBride, a great friend who introduced us to the Beauty Foundation and who continues to work, walk, and raise both funds and awareness for cancer research, treatment, and cures.

And to anyone whose name might be missing, we both thank you for being there for us; while you may not be on this list, you'll always be in our hearts.

Marybeth Adds

On a personal note, I would like to thank my "baby" Christopher and "big boy" Brian for being the best boys a mom could have; my dad, John V. Maher, for showing me through example how to face cancer with courage, strength, and humor; my mom, Veronica Maher; sister Christine Kessler; brothers John and Michael Maher; sisters- and brothers-in-law; nieces and nephews; aunts and uncles; cousins; and family friends for their cards, good wishes, and ever-present support. My mother- and father-in-law, Vincenza and Vincent Maida, for holding my family together as we dealt with this disease; Vinny Maida for holding my hand as I awaited surgery; Caren Maher for putting me back together when I was literally falling apart; Stephanie Escandon, for rides to the doctor, talks on the phone, wonderful lunches, and ready support; and Janis Wilkins for never leaving me alone in a hospital room.

I would also like to express deep appreciation to my oncologist, Dr. John Sierocki, for his compassion, dedication, and brilliance. Great thanks as well to plastic surgeon Dr. Lloyd Gayle and his nurse Pamela Messina, for taking my battered body under their wing and giving me back a figure to love.

Debbie Adds

I would like to thank my three beautiful daughters, Mika, Natasha, and Katarina Cucullo, who have given me the true understanding of love at its deepest level; my parents, Mary Lou and Fred Kiederer, who have cared for and supported my family during the best and worst of times; Jan and Rob Laquidara, who traveled hours and late nights to help during Bobby's illnesses; Silvia Liehn, who held the family together when I was working or at the hospital for hours each day with two small children to care for at home; and my sister, Laurie, and brother, Glenn, and their families, who were always there to lend a hand or an ear whenever needed. To Danielle Alexander and Kristin and Brian Leschke—remember to carry your mother's memory and love in your heart always. To my college roommates—Lois, Patty, Julie, Bridgit, Jodi, and Julie—the years shared with Sue were incredibly special—memories made to be cherished for a lifetime.

INDEX

Academy of Medical Acupuncturists, 195
Accessories, 111–15
  hats, 120–22
Aches and pains, 139–45
  diagnosis, 140–41
  intervention, 141–44
Acidophilus, 167
Acne, 62, 91–92
Acupressure, 188–89
Acupuncture, 186–88
Acupuncturists, 194–96
Alcohol, 155, 176
Allergic reactions, 93–94
Alternative medicine, 183–201
  acupuncture, 186–88
  easing dis-ease, 197–200
  finding caregivers, 194–97
  massage therapy, 188–92
  music therapy, 193–94
  websites, 200–201
American Cancer Society, 29–30,
  129, 180
American Dietetic Association
  (ADA), 180
American Institute for Cancer Research (AICR), 180
Anastasia of Beverly Hills. See
  Soare, Anastasia
Antianxiety drugs, 136–37
Antiemetics, 157
Anti-inflammatory drugs, 156
Anti-inflammatory foods, 165

Antinausea drugs, 101
Antioxidants, in moisturizers, 69
Anti-seizure drugs, 156
Anxiety, 207–8
Appearance, 27–28
  acceptance of, 233–35
Artificial devices, for pain, 144
Ashiness (ashy skin), 89, 120
Asking for help, 126–27
Astringents, 70–71
Atlas, 229–33
Attire. See Clothing

Baldness, 34–36, 53. See also Hair
  and hair loss
  transitioning back from, 56–57
  when shedding starts, 54–55
Band and coil, 48–49
Bangs, and wigs, 44
Baseball caps, 54
Baths, 67–68
Bathwater, 68
Benson, Herbert, 214
Berkowitz, Leah
  accessories, 112–15, 121, 122
  biographical sketch, 1
  fashion and clothing, 102
    dresses, 108–9
    fabric, 115
    proper fit, 118
    skin tone and color,
      119–20
  parting wisdom, 251

Bjerke, Eivind
  baldness, 54
  biographical sketch, 1
  hair care, 56, 59
  parting wisdom, 248
  wigs, 37, 38–39, 43, 44
Bladder infections, 166–67
Blandi, Oscar
  baldness, 54
  biographical sketch, 2
  positive attitude, 253
  wigs, 38, 43
Blood deficiency headaches, 153
Blushes, 79–80
Body
  cleansing, 67–68
  moisturizing, 69–70
Body aches and pains, 139–45
  diagnosis, 140–41
  intervention, 141–44
Body butters, 69–70
Body shape, 101, 116–19
  clothing and, 108–9
  excessive thinness, 117–19
Bone aches and pains. *See* Aches
    and pains
Bone density and osteoporosis,
    167–69
Bow, the, 49–50
Bragagnini, Amy
  biographical sketch, 2
  diet, 145, 166, 171, 173–74,
    177–80
    advance preparation,
      171–72
  exercise, 177
  parting wisdom, 246
  water intake, 145
Breakfast at Tiffany's (movie), 111
Brushes, makeup, 79–80
Burke, Michele
  biographical sketch, 2
  face and skin, 63–64
    acne, 91–92
    cleansers, 66, 67
    moisturizers, 69
    toners, 71
  focus on key feature, 74–75, 109
  makeup, 95, 96–97

  blushes, 79
  concealers, 78–79
  dark circles under eyes,
    87–88
  eyebrows, 84–85
  eye color tint, 86–87
  eyelashes, 83
  eye shadow, 81
  foundations, 76, 78
  lipsticks, 80
  parting wisdom, 252
  positive attitude, 96–97

Caffeine, 137, 176
Calcium, 168
Canned foods, 179
Canzone, Sandy, 134
  biographical sketch, 2
  diet and eating right, 172–75,
    178
  drowsiness/insomnia, 146,
    147–48
  headaches, 153
  herbal remedies, 133, 148
  hot flashes, 165–66
  integrative (Eastern)
    approaches, 184, 198, 199
    acupuncture, 187, 195–96
    massage, 191, 192
    music therapy, 193
  nausea, 157, 158–59
  parting wisdom, 256
  vaginal dryness, 170
Caps, 54
  for wigs, 41–42
Caputo, Thomas
  biographical sketch, 2
  parting wisdom, 256
  sexual side effects of
    chemotherapy, 164, 167,
    169–70
Chamomile, 90
Chapman, Cheryl
  asking for help, 126–27, 247
  biographical sketch, 3
  massage therapy, 166, 188–92
  music therapy, 193–94
Chapsticks, 80
Chemotherapy, 135–39

body beautiful, 159–60
changes to taste, 178–79
eating after infusion, 174–76
eating before infusion, 172–74
sexual side effects, 161–70
  bone density/osteoporosis,
    167–69
  hot flashes, 165–66
  infections, 166–67
  sex, 169–70
side effects, 139–59
  bone/muscle aches and
    pains, 139–45
  constipation/diarrhea,
    145–46
  drowsiness/insomnia,
    146–50
  fatigue, 150–52
  headaches, 152–54
  nausea, 157–59
  numbness/neuropathy,
    154–57
  websites, 160
Chi (qi) energy, 186–87
Clothing (fashion), 99–124
  accessories, 111–15, 120–22
  body shape and, 101, 116–19
  colors of, 105–6, 119–20
  fabric choices, 115–16
  fit of, 106–8, 118
  illusion and distraction, 109–10
  projecting inner beauty, 122–24
  proportions of, 108–9
  skin tone and, 119–20
  survivors' stories, 99–100
  undergarments, 104–5
Coconut oil, 142–43, 170
Coconut water, 175
Cold caps, 35
Color
  of clothing, 105–6, 119–20
  of wigs, 43
Concealers, 78–79
Constipation, 145–46
Consultations with doctors,
  130–31
Cortisol, and massages, 192
Cosmetics, 27–32, 73–88
  blushes, 79–80

concealers, 78–79
eyebrows, 84–86
eye color tint, 86–87
eyes, 81–82
foundations, 75–78
lashes, 81–84
lipsticks, 80
skin-related side effects, 87–97
sunken eyes, 87
websites, 97–98
Costume jewelry, 113–15
Cotton clothing, 115–16
Counselors, 230–31, 247
Crisis as an opportunity, 224–26
Custom wigs, 45–47
Cut, of wigs, 43–45

Dairy, 174–75, 178
Dark circles under eyes, 87–88
Dark spots, 92–93
Dates, 173–74
DeAngelo, Christine
  biographical sketch, 3
  fashion and clothing, 103, 248
    dresses, 109
    fabric choices, 115
    fit, 107
    layering, 118
    skin tone and, 119–20
    undergarments, 105
DeMarco, Francine
  accessories, 112, 114, 121–22
  biographical sketch, 3
  fashion and clothing, 101, 102,
    109–11
    color, 105–6
    dresses, 119
    loungewear, 115–16
    proportions, 108
    skin tone and, 119–20
    undergarments, 104
  hope and passion, 248–49
  on Marilyn Monroe, 123
DeMontpensier, Louis Philippe
  biographical sketch, 3–4
  face and skin, 66, 68, 69, 95
  fashion and clothing, 103
  makeup, 74, 75, 78, 80–85, 87, 96
  parting wisdom, 251

Denial, 232–33
Dental care, 179
Deodorant soaps, 68
Depression, 143, 232
Diarrhea, 145–46
Dibsie, Krista
  biographical sketch, 4
  face and skin, 65, 68, 90
  lipsticks, 80
  parting wisdom, 250
DiCecca, Rick
  biographical sketch, 4
  hair loss, 36, 54
  makeup, 73–75, 77, 83, 87, 91
  parting wisdom, 254
Diet, 171–82
  advance preparation, 171–72
  changes to taste, 178–79
  eating after infusion, 174–76
  eating before infusion, 172–74
  fruits and vegetables, 179–80
  websites, 180, 182
  weight gain, 176–77
  weight loss, 178
Diflucan, 167
Dis-ease, 197–200
Disposable needles, for acupunc-
    ture, 188
Dress. See Clothing
Dresses, 108–9, 118–19
Drowsiness, 146–50
Drugstores, 67, 76
Dry brain, 153
Dry mouth, 176
Dry skin, 63

Earrings, 112
Eastern (integrative) medicine,
    183–201
  acupuncture, 186–88
  easing dis-ease, 197–200
  finding caregivers, 194–97
  massage therapy, 188–92
  music therapy, 193–94
  websites, 200–201
Eating right, 171–82
  advance preparation, 171–72
  changes to taste, 178–79
  eating after infusion, 174–76

eating before infusion, 172–74
  fruits and vegetables, 179–80
  websites, 180, 182
  weight gain, 176–77
  weight loss, 178
Energy journals, 152
Estrogen, 162–64
Ethical wills, 227–29
Exercise, 145, 150–51, 158, 177,
    236
Exfoliation, 70–71
Eyebrows, 63, 84–86
  four-step process for drawing,
    85–86
Eye color tint, 63, 86–87
Eyelashes, 63, 81–84
Eye makeup, 81–82
Eyes, sunken, 87
Eye shadow, 81, 82

Fabrics, 107, 115–16
Face. See also Makeup
  cleansing, 66–67
  moisturizing, 68–69
  peels, 70–71
  side effects, 63
Facial massages, 90
Faith, 203–41, 249–50
  acceptance of appearance,
    233–35
  achieving oneness, 213–24
  ancient texts, 236–37
  ethical wills, 227–29
  a family affair, 226–29
  meditation, 213–18
  prayer of life, 237–39
  "thy will be done," 218–24
  viewing crisis as an opportunity,
    224–26
  websites, 240–41
  what to do, 209–12
False eyelashes, 82–83
Family, support from, 126–27,
    226–29, 248
Fashion (clothing), 99–124
  accessories, 111–15, 120–22
  body shape and, 101, 116–19
  colors of, 105–6, 119–20
  fabric choices, 115–16

fit of, 106–8, 118
illusion and distraction,
  109–10
projecting inner beauty, 122–24
proportions of, 108–9
skin tone and, 119–20
survivors' stories, 99–100
undergarments, 104–5
Fashion Week (New York City),
  xIII–xIv
Fatigue, 150–52
Fears, 205, 207–8
Fiber, in your diet, 145
Figs, 173–74
Fit of clothing, 106–8, 118
Fluid intake, 145, 153, 175–76
Flushing/redness, 63, 90–91
Foundation garments, 104–5
Foundation makeup, 75–78
Friends, support from, 126–27,
  226–29, 248
Fruits and vegetables, 172, 180

Gayle, Lloyd, 4, 250–51
Geary, Deann
  biographical sketch, 4
  hair loss, 34–35
  hair styles, 58, 59
  support network, 248
  wigs, 36, 37, 39–47
Gedeon, Harvey
  biographical sketch, 5
  face and skin, 65–67
    cleansers, 66, 67
    hyperpigmentation, 93
    rashes, 94
    redness/flushing, 90
    sunscreens, 69
Gibson, Amy
  biographical sketch, 5
  hair loss, 35, 38
  hair styles, 58–59
  parting wisdom, 246
  scalp care, 55
  scarves for turbans, 47
  wigs, 41, 43, 44
Gilson, Noah
  biographical sketch, 5
  headaches, 153

numbness/neuropathy, 154–55
  parting wisdom, 252
Ginger tea, 157
Glycolic acids, 70–71
Goji berry extract, 90
Gransil, 77
Green tea, 147, 175

Hair and hair loss, 33–59
  caring for your scalp, 55
  fear of baldness, 34–36
  side effects, 34, 35–36
  survivors' stories, 33–34
  transitioning back from bald-
    ness, 56–57
  T-shirt wrap for, 53
  turbans for, 47–53
  websites, 59–60
  when shedding starts, 54–55
  wigs for, 36–47
Hair coloring, 56–57
Hair conditioners, 56
Hairdressers, 57–59
Half bow, 52
Haloxyl, 92
Handbags, 112, 114
Handmade wig caps, 42
Hats, 54, 120–22
Headaches, 152–54
  acupressure for, 188–89
Heat, for aches and pains, 142
Hepburn, Audrey, 111
Herbal remedies, 132–33, 148
Hives, 93–94
Holistic medicine. See Integrative
  approach
Hope, 248–49
Hot flashes, 162, 165–66
Hot spicy foods, 166
Human hair wigs, 39–40
Hydration, 145, 153, 175–76
Hydrochinone, 92
Hydrocolators, 142–43
Hyperpigmentation, 92–93

Inner strength, 205–7. See also
  Faith
Insomnia, 146–50
Insurance, for wigs, 40–41

Integrative approach, 183–201
  acupuncture, 186–88
  easing dis-ease, 197–200
  finding caregivers, 194–97
  massage therapy, 188–92
  music therapy, 193–94
  websites, 200–201
Internet research, 129–30
Iridescence, 77
Isoflavones, 166
Isolation, 249

Jewelry, 112–15
Johnson, Betsey, xiii–xvi
  biographical sketch, 5
  fashion and clothing, 101,
    103–4, 108
    color, 105, 109, 118
    fabric choices, 115
  support network, 246–47
Jojoba beads, 71

Kobeisy, Ahmed Nezar
  acceptance of appearance, 234,
    235
  biographical sketch, 6
  depression, 232
  keeping the faith, 208, 219, 222,
    224
  parting wisdom, 245–46

Lavender, 90
Layering clothing, 118
Lean meats, 178
Libido, 169–70
Lidoderm, 142
Lip glosses, 80
Lips, dry, 63
Lipsticks, 80
Liquor, 155, 176
Look Good Feel Better Founda-
  tion, 29–30
Loupuchin, Theresa, 30
  baths, 68
  biographical sketch, 6
  face and skin, 64–67, 69–73
    astringents, 71
    cleansers, 66–67
    moisturizers, 69–70

  redness, 90, 92
  sun protection, 72–73
  makeup, 95, 96–97
    blushes, 79
    eye color tint, 86–87
    eyelashes, 82–83
    foundations, 75–76, 78, 92, 93
    lipsticks, 80
    sallow skin, 89
    sunken eyes, 87
  parting wisdom, 256
  scalp care, 55
  scarves, 47–48

MacDonald, Gayle
  biographical sketch, 6–7
  massage therapy, 156–57, 166,
    189–90, 192, 196–97
  parting wisdom, 249
Mahanarayan Oil, 192
Makeup, 27–32, 73–88
  blushes, 79–80
  concealers, 78–79
  eyebrows, 84–86
  eye color tint, 86–87
  eyes, 81–82
  foundations, 75–78
  lashes, 81–84
  lipsticks, 80
  skin-related side effects, 87–97
  sunken eyes, 87
  websites, 97–98
Makeup brushes, 79–80
Massages, 152–53, 156–57, 188–92
Massages therapists, 196–97
Matte lipsticks, 80
Medical team, 132–35
  selecting your, 129–32
Meditation, 213–18
Medley, Patricia S. (Pastor Pat)
  biographical sketch, 7
  keeping the faith, 209–10,
    219–21, 225–26, 233–34,
    236–38, 253
  parting wisdom, 253
Melanin, excessive, 95–96
Menopause, hot flashes, 162,
  165–66
Microabrasion, 70–71

Milk cleansers, 66
Milkshakes, 178
Mineral powders, 77
Minerals, 180
Minocin, 90
Moisturizers, 68–71
    body, 69–70
    face, 68–69
Monroe, Marilyn, 123
Morris, Robert Lee, 7, 113, 255
Mouth care, 179
Mouth sores, 179
Murad, Howard
    biographical sketch, 7
    face and skin, 64–65, 69–72
        acne, 91
        exfoliants, 71
        lip ointments, 80
        moisturizers, 69, 70
        rashes, 94
        redness/flushing, 90
        sunburn-type pain, 94–95
        sunscreen, 72, 92
    isolation, 249
Muscle aches and pains, 139–45
    diagnosis, 140–41
    intervention, 141–44
Music therapy, 193–94

Naps (napping), 149–50
National Certification Commis-
    sion for Acupuncture and
    Oriental Medicine
    (NCCAOM), 195
Natural fabrics, 115–16
Nausea, 157–59
    acupuncture for, 186
Neuroblockades, 143–44
Neuropathy, 95, 154–57
New York City Fashion Week,
    xiii–xiv
New York Times, 244–45
Nies, John
    biographical sketch, 7–8
    exercise, 150–51
    keeping the faith, 250
    visualization, 149
North American Neurological In-
    vasive Society, 144

Numbness, 154–57
Nurses, oncology, 133–34, 136–37
Nutmeg, 148
Nutrition. See Diet

Oncologists, 132–35
    selecting your, 129–32
Oncology massage, 188–92
Oncology nurses, 133–34, 136–37
Oncology team, 132–35
    selecting your, 129–32
Oneness, achieving, 213–24
    meditation, 213–18
Oribe
    biographical sketch, 8
    hair care, 56–57
    hair loss, 55
    hair styles, 57
    parting wisdom, 252
    scalp care, 55
    scarves for turbans, 47
    wigs, 36–39, 42, 44–45
Osteoporosis, 167–69

Pain medications, 141–42
Pains, 139–45
    diagnosis, 140–41
    intervention, 141–44
Paul, Saint, 233–34
Pedialyte, 175
Peels, 70–71
Peirano, Daniel (Father Dan)
    biographical sketch, 8–9
    keeping the faith, 208, 211,
        222–23, 230, 239
    parting wisdom, 248
Peripheral neuropathy, 154–57
Personal Care Products Council,
    29–30
Perspiration, and wig caps, 41
Pigmentation, uneven, 63, 92–93
Pimples, 62, 91–92
Poppy seeds, 148
Positive attitude, 18, 96–97,
    218–19, 247, 253
Pramagel, 94–95
Pramosone lotion, 94–95
Prayer of life, 237–39
Projecting inner beauty, 122–24

Proportions of clothing, 108–9
Psychiatrists, 230–31
Psychologists, 230–31

Qi (chi) energy, 186–87
Q-tips, 95

Rahman Kahn, Abdur
  biographical sketch, 5–6
  keeping the faith, 211, 222, 223,
    227, 234, 235, 256
Raisins, 173–74
Rashes, 63, 93–94
Redness/flushing, 63, 90–91
Reflexology, 156–57, 166
Reiki, 156–57
Relaxation Response (Benson), 214
Religious faith. *See* Faith
Rhythmic breathing, 215–16
Roos, Jonathan
  biographical sketch, 9
  keeping the faith, 210, 211–12,
    220, 226–28, 230, 235, 237,
    238–39
  parting wisdom, 254
Rosacea, 90–91
Rosette, 51

Saint Laurent, Yves, 103
Salicylic acid, 90, 91
Sallowness (sallow skin), 63,
    88–89, 119–20
Salt intake, 172, 176–77
Sarna lotion, 94–95
Scalp care, 55
Scarves, 47–53, 122
  band and coil option, 48–49
  the basics, 48
  the bow, 49–50
  half bow, 52
  rosette, 51
  square knot, 50
Schneider, Samuel
  biographical sketch, 9
  keeping the faith, 206, 220–21,
    223–25, 227, 229, 231–34
  parting wisdom, 255
Sea-Bands, 157–58, 188

Sedatives, 136–37
Self-advocacy, 248
Self-affirmations, 218–19
Self-denial, 232–33
Sex drive, 169–70
Sexual side effects of chemother-
    apy, 161–70
  bone density/osteoporosis,
    167–69
  hot flashes, 165–66
  infections, 166–67
  sex, 169–70
Shiatsu, 166
Shingles, 94
Shoes, 112
Showers, 68
Side effects
  chemotherapy, 139–59
    bone/muscle aches and
      pains, 139–45
    constipation/diarrhea,
      145–46
    drowsiness/insomnia,
      146–50
    fatigue, 150–52
    headaches, 152–54
    nausea, 157–59
    numbness/neuropathy,
      154–57
  hair loss, 34, 35–36
  sexual, 161–70
    bone density/osteoporosis,
      167–69
    hot flashes, 165–66
    infections, 166–67
    sex, 169–70
  skin-related, 62–64, 88–97
    acne, 62, 91–92
    ashiness, 89
    excessive melanin, 95–96
    neuropathy, 95
    rashes, 63, 93–94
    redness/flushing, 63, 90–91
    sallowness, 63, 88–89
    sunburn-type pain, 63,
      94–95
    uneven pigmentation, 63,
      92–93

Sizes, clothing, 106–8
Skin (skin care), 61–73. *See also*
    Makeup
    cleansing your body, 67–68
    cleansing your face, 66–67
    clothing choices and, 119–20
    moisturizing your body, 69–70
    moisturizing your face, 68–69
    peels, 70–71
    side effects, 62–64, 88–97
        acne, 62, 91–92
        ashiness, 89
        excessive melanin, 95–96
        neuropathy, 95
        rashes, 63, 93–94
        redness/flushing, 63, 90–91
        sallowness, 63, 88–89
        sunburn-type pain, 63,
            94–95
        uneven pigmentation, 63,
            92–93
    survivors' stories, 61–62
    websites, 97–98
Skin Cancer Foundation, 72
Skin cells, 64–65
Sleep, insomnia, 146–50
Sleeping pills, 149
Sleep patterns, 147–48
Soaps, 66–68
Soare, Anastasia (Anastasia of
    Beverly Hills)
    biographical sketch, 1
    dark circles under eyes, 87
    eyebrow stencils, 84
    eye color tint, 86
    makeup, 74, 95
    parting wisdom, 246
Society for Integrative Oncology,
    194–95
Society for Oncology Massage, 196
Sodium, 172, 176–77
Soups, 172–74
Spellmeyer, Kurt
    biographical sketch, 9
    keeping the faith, 206, 210, 212,
        215–17, 219, 221–22, 225
    parting wisdom, 251
Spicy foods, 166

Spirituality and faith, 203–41,
    249–50
    acceptance of appearance, 233–35
    achieving oneness, 213–24
    ancient texts, 236–37
    ethical wills, 227–29
    a family affair, 226–29
    meditation, 213–18
    prayer of life, 237–39
    "thy will be done," 218–24
    viewing crisis as an opportunity,
        224–26
    websites, 240–41
    what to do, 209–12
Sports bras, 104
Square knot, 50
Staats, Peter
    acupuncture, 187–88
    biographical sketch, 9–10
    pain management, 141, 143–44,
        254
Stencils, 84–86
Steroids, 62, 101
Stress, and pain, 143
Sugar intake, 155
Sunburn-type pain, 63, 94–95
Sun exposure, 72–73
Sunken eyes, 87
Sunscreens, 69, 72–73, 80
Supplements, 180
Support groups, 129–30, 230,
    231–32
Support network, 126–27, 226–29,
    248
Sweat glands, 64–65
Symptoms, treating your, 134–35
Synthetic wigs, 39–40

Taste buds, 178–79
Tea tree oil, 179
TENS (transcutaneous electrical
    nerve stimulation), 154
Tetracycline, 90
Thinness, excessive, 117–19
"Thy will be done," 218–24
Tight clothing, 119
Titanium dioxide, 69, 73
Toners, 70–71

Torpey, Brian
  aches and pains, 140–42
  biographical sketch, 10
  bone density, 168–69
  neuropathy, 155–56
  parting wisdom, 247
Traumeel, 142–43
Trigger points, 187
T-shirt wrap, 53–54
Turbans, 47–53
  band and coil option, 48–49
  the basics, 48
  the bow, 49
  half bow, 52
  rosette, 51
  square knot, 50

Undergarments, 104–5
UPF (Ultraviolet Protection Factor), 72
Urine color, 176

Vaginal dilators, 170
Vaginal dryness, 169–70
Vaginal moisturizers, 170
Visualization, 148–49
Vitamin A-rich vegetables, for sallow skin, 89
Vitamin B6, 156
Vitamin B12, 156
Vitamin C, in moisturizers, 69
Vitamin D, 168
Vitamin E, 170
Vitamins, 180
Viviscal, 55

Wardrobe. See Clothing
Warrior image, 29
Water intake, 145, 153, 175–76
Websites (Web research), 129–30
  chemotherapy, 160
  diet, 180, 182
  hair, 59–60
  integrative medicine, 200–201
  keeping the faith, 240–41
  skin care and makeup, 97–98
Weight gain, 101, 176–77
Weight loss, 117–19, 178
Weinrib, Joann, 215

aches and pains, 142–43
biographical sketch, 10
diet and eating right, 172, 174, 175–77
fatigue, 151–52
headaches, 152–53
insomnia, 147–49
keeping the faith, 249
supplements, 180
treating the symptom, 134
Wexler, Patricia
  biographical sketch, 10
  face and skin, 65, 69–73, 89–94, 96
  parting wisdom, 253–54
  showers, 68
Whole grain breads, 172
Wigs, 36–47
  caps, 41–42
  choosing, 38–39
  color of, 43
  cut of, 43–45
  insurance for, 40–41
  measuring custom, 45–47
  synthetic vs. human, 39–40
Wig salons, 57–59
Wills, ethical, 227–29
Witch hazel, 55
Wrap dresses, 119
Wright, Leonard
  biographical sketch, 10
  fitness program, 151
  integrative (Eastern)
    approaches, 183–85, 198–99
    acupuncture, 186–88, 194–95
  Internet research, 130
  meditation, 213–14, 217–18
  mouth sores, 179
  nausea, 157–58
  open dialogue with medical team, 132
  parting wisdom, 250
  second opinions, 128–29

Yeast infections, 166–67
Yellow eye color tint, 63, 86–87
Yoga, 151

Zinc oxide, 69, 73